FEELING GOOD LIKE I SHOULD

HOW TO SLEEP BETTER TO IMPROVE YOUR MIND, BODY, AND LIFE

ALEX LUTON

LEGAL NOTICE

This book is copyright protected. It is only for personal use. You cannot amend, distribute, sell, use, quote or paraphrase any part, or the content within this book, without the consent of the author or publisher.

Please note the information contained within this document is for educational and entertainment purposes only. All effort has been executed to present accurate, up to date, reliable, complete information. No warranties of any kind are declared or implied. Readers acknowledge that the author is not engaged in the rendering of legal, financial, medical or profes-sional advice. The content within this book has been derived from various sources. Please consult a licensed professional before attempting any tech-niques outlined in this book.

By reading this document, the reader agrees that under no circumstances is the author responsible for any losses, direct or indirect, that are incurred as a result of the use of the information contained within this document, including, but not limited to, errors, omissions, or inaccuracies.

DISCLAIMER NOTICE

result of the use of the information contained within this document, including, but not limited to, errors, omissions, or inaccuracies.

CONTENTS

Legal Notice 1

Disclaimer Notice 3

Introduction 7

Chapter 1 - The Function of Sleep 11

Chapter 2 - The Body's Internal Clock 25

Chapter 3 - Sleep Debt 33

Chapter 4 - Quality vs. Quantity Sleep 45

Chapter 5 - Insomnia 53

Chapter 6 - Sleep Disturbances 59

Chapter 7 - Creating a Sleep Sanctuary 73

Chapter 8 - Sleep Hygiene and How to Get 87
Better Sleep

Chapter 9 - Fall Asleep Faster 113

Chapter 10 - Sleep Therapy 131

Conclusion 141

References 145

INTRODUCTION

Are you not sleeping through the night, unable to fall asleep quickly, and feeling exhausted throughout the day? Sound familiar? Chances are this describes a typical night and day for you. Millions of people struggle with sleep. Just because this is a common struggle does not make it any easier.

Not getting enough sleep does more than just make us more irritable and emotional. Being unable to concentrate, remain awake, and make simple choices throughout the day are all also side effects of poor sleep that can have negative consequences in other areas of our lives. Unfortunately, many fail to make this connection. When we are irritable, our relationships suffer; when we are unable to stay awake, we miss out on being active in our lives. When we make poor choices or careless mistakes, our jobs and school life are negatively affected.

This is not to say there has not been an effort to try to correct these side effects. May reach for energy drinks or coffee regularly to keep themselves alert and attentive. Others try sleep medication to get the right hours of sleep at night. However, despite these efforts, your sleep is not improving. This is because most of the efforts people take to improve their sleep are only bandages that mask the real issues.

To finally overcome the struggles you have been having with sleep, you need to look at sleep from a new perspective. You need to understand that finding quick solutions to get to sleep faster will only temporarily help you improve your issues. Why many continue to have issues with their sleep is not just because they do not want to sleep, it is because they do not have the right mindset to encourage sleep.

As a sleep specialist, I have spent over 25 years researching and helping thousands of individuals overcome many sleep disorders. The earlier years of my work caused me to experience firsthand the negative effects of losing sleep. Long hours at the office, frequent trips to conferences, and staying up late to relax begin to cause my work to suffer. I had to take my own advice and make sleep a priority. I had to change my mindset of looking at sleep as something that is nice to enjoy to seeing it as an important factor that transforms my happiness and way of living.

In this book, I have compiled over two decades of learning to help you tackle and finally get the sleep you need. You will fully understand how poor sleep habits are causing you to not just feel more tired during the day but putting you at risk for more serious complications. There is information that discusses the most common sleep disturbances and disorders that you will want to further discuss with your doctor. Parents and caregivers will find beneficial information regarding not just how they can improve their sleep for themselves but for their children as well.

You will learn about the most important factors for setting up the right sleep environment so that you look forward to getting into bed each night. There is a plethora of information covering your daily activities and changes to implement to promote a better night's sleep. On top of these environmental and lifestyle changes, you will find plenty of useful techniques that can help you combat stress and anxiety to fall asleep faster. Instead of letting sleepless nights contribute to your sleep loss, you will have go-to methods to help you sleep better and longer.

The information in this book will provide you with alternative ways to correct your sleep problems. You do not need to rely on sleep aids to fall asleep or caffeine to stay awake during the day. You will be able to make simple changes and experiment with other options to allow your body to naturally fall into sleep mode and shift into alert mode when it is appropriate. More importantly, you see what a difference a good night's sleep actually makes. Your mood, health, and happiness will all take an upward swing.

Feeling exhausted day after day is no way to live a fulfilling life: it is also not something you should just accept and live with. There are effective ways to naturally sleep better—and you are about to learn them. If you are tired of being tired, it is time to take control of your sleep and experience the bliss of getting restorative, rejuvenating, and consistent quality sleep.

CHAPTER 1 - THE FUNCTION OF SLEEP

Skipping out on sleep may seem like a harmless act, but the short and long-term effects can be substantial and impact every area of your life. Most individuals think sleep is a luxury. When they can sleep they do; if they do not get enough, they just accept that as their normal. The normal being a feeling of tiredness the next day, being irritable, or just side effects they deal with after a poor night's sleep. These minor infractions only scratch the surface as to how sleep impacts our health, happiness, and life. If you struggle with sleep, you need to first understand why it is important to get the right sleep every night and the vital roles it plays in keeping our body and mind function at an optimal level.

. . .

Sleep Physiology

When we sleep we are in a state of unawareness. Sleep is a crucial time for our body and mind to rejuvenate and reset. While it appears that nothing is going on when we sleep, our bodies are going through many processes. This includes organizing and storing information, healing and producing new cells, as well as giving us uninterrupted time to gain clarity and more energy for the following day.

We sleep in two different phases—rapid eye movement sleep (REM) and non-rapid eye movement sleep (Non-REM). Each of these phases contributes to how beneficial our sleep is as well as how many hours of sleep we enjoy.

REM Sleep

REM sleep gets its name from the presence of rapid eye movement, where you can see the eyes moving under the lids as you are sleeping. This occurs because our brain activity increases while we are in this stage. This also causes our heart rate and breathing to become slightly irregular. Since our brains are on high alert at this time, we are easily woken. It is also during this stage that we remember the dreams that occur.

REM sleep is an important stage because when we

enter into REM sleep, the learning and memory areas of our brain are stimulated. It is also a time where the brain neurons are formulating stronger connections that impact our overall health and happiness. REM sleep occurs within 90 minutes of falling asleep. During the first cycle we only spend 10 minutes in REM sleep, but the longer we sleep, the longer our REM sleep gets. Infants spend a significant part of their time sleeping in the REM stage; as we age, and especially in older age, we spend less and less time experiencing REM sleep.

Non-REM Sleep

Non-REM sleep consists of four different stages. The first is typically the shortest, only lasting about 10 minutes and starts from the time you fall asleep. The second stage tends to be the longest lasting: up to an hour after stage one. Here, the muscles are relaxed and slow-wave activity occurs. In stage three of non-REM sleep, we are in the deepest sleep. This stage can last from 20 to 40 minutes. During each stage of non-REM sleep, everything begins to slow down. Brain activity continually slows, your heart rate decreases, breathing is more relaxed, and there is no body movement unless you are in stage three. During stage four, non-REM sleep is when most of the restorative processes take place. Muscle healing, tissue, and cell growth occurs, and energy is refueled.

Stage three and four of non-REM sleep is when we are in our deepest sleep. While dreams do occur during this stage, they are not remembered as they are not stored as memories in the brain.

Sleep Effects

Sleep has a direct and indirect impact on all functions in the body. It can also affect external areas of our lives. It is important to understand that many negative side effects of losing sleep can take years to develop, but even the short-term effects can cause serious impairments.

Immune System

Well-rested individuals tend to get sick less often. This is because of the complex relationship that sleep and the immune system have. The immune system, as we know, is responsible for warding off infections and protecting the body from viruses and harmful pathogens. When our immune system is in optimal shape, it can fight off attacks from foreign pathogens and can respond quickly to injury (Suni, 2020). For the immune system to function properly, it needs time to store information about the antigens uncovered from encountering pathogens. Antigens are parts of the pathogens that trigger the immune response; if the antigen has been detected before, the body calls upon the proper defense to quickly rid the harmful intruders. If the antigen has not been detected before, the immune system copies it to properly attack it when it enters the body again.

Each antigen is stored in the immune system's memory, much like skills and information can be stored in the brain and retrieved at a later time. The immune system utilizes the time we sleep to organize and properly store antigen information.

It is also during sleep, specifically deep sleep, when the body can redirect energy to the immune system to heal and restore damaged cells and tissues. This energy is also used by the immune system to perform crucial tasks like hormone production and triggering inflammation necessary to keep the rest of the body function efficiently.

Hormones

Stress hormones, like cortisol, are released when we are alert or when the brain signals that we should be alert. When we skip out on sleep, we produce more cortisol than we need. Melatonin, a crucial hormone that promotes sleep, is also produced while we sleep. If we stay up watching television or reading with the lights on, we halt the production of melatonin, making it more difficult to fall asleep. Light exposure sends signals to the brain to stop melatonin production and triggers stimulating hormones like cortisol.

Health Conditions

If we do not get enough sleep, we put ourselves at risk for a wide range of serious health conditions. Lack of sleep can negatively affect our respiratory system, cardiovascular system, and blood pressure. Since sleep is responsible for keeping our hormones in check, when these become out of balance—like cortisol—our blood pressure increases. Higher blood pressure leads to heart problems and other disorders that affect us for the long-term.

Mental health is also significantly impacted. Not getting enough sleep makes us feel more tired and unable to complete everything we need to get done. This inability to have the energy to do what we are capable of can diminish how we view ourselves. Poor health—that is a by-product of not enough sleep—also causes us to stress and feel more anxious.

SLEEP AND COGNITIVE FUNCTION

When you do not get enough sleep, you quickly suffer from the effects: inability to concentrate, logically think through decisions, miss important details, and are less productive. These short-term effects may have instant consequences, but there is much more that deteriorates with our cognitive function when we do not get enough sleep. When you get enough sleep, you will react to situations with clarity, you can focus for longer periods of time, and you are more alert.

Memory

Memory is affected by sleep when the blood vessels in the brain begin to narrow. Less blood flow is circulating to and from the brain which is depriving the cells in the brain of essential oxygen and sugar.

Sleep is also the time when information retained through the day is transformed into a memory, so that it can be recalled again at a later time. This directly affects our ability to learn, to make use of new skills, and process information we need to get enough sleep so that the neurons in the brain can function optimally. When the neurons are overworked and are not given enough time to properly process information received in the day, we are unable to access the information for later use.

Different types of memories rely on different stages of sleep for proper storage in the brain. Declarative memories—fact-based knowledge—requires adequate REM sleep. Procedural memories—those that relate to how to do something—requires enough

REM and non-REM sleep (Healthy Sleep, n.d.). REM and non-REM sleep are crucial for us to be able to consolidate different types of information—visual, motor, audible—and the length of these sleep stages also impact our ability to retrieve the information properly to use when needed. Getting enough REM sleep is vital for us to be able to access the information we have already learned.

The effect sleep has on our mood can also hinder our ability to remember things. When we do not get enough sleep and are more on edge emotionally, we are not able to properly acquire new information. Emotionally-charged memories also require REM sleep for proper storage. When we are unable to store these types of memories or access them when similar situations arise in our lives, we will not know how to handle them properly. This can result in repeated, undesirable behaviors.

Decision-Making

Sleep plays an important role in the decision-making process. To be able to access stored information and make appropriate decisions, we need to be able to plan accordingly and assess the situation clearly. When we are not well-rested, our judgment is impaired, and we may not choose the correct behaviors in certain situations. This is because the neurons in the brain are not able to send the right signals; the muscle and organs in the body are not able to receive the correct signals either because they also become fatigued.

This is why we are more prone to accidents, minor and serious, when we are fatigued. Our brains simply cannot function fast enough to stop or prevent accidents from occurring.

Brain Degeneration

Individuals who sleep poorly tend to have a higher deposit of beta-amyloid, a protein deposit. This build-up of beta-amyloid has been linked to significant decline of memory that results in dementia and further develops into more serious brain degenerative diseases like Alzheimer's disease and Parkinson's disease (Smith, 2018).

What is more concerning is, the parts of the brain that are impacted first from lack of sleep are the same areas that trigger deep and restorative sleep. Losing sleep not only hampers our brain health, the areas of the brain it affects first contributes to further degeneration.

.

. . .

WEIGHT

If you struggle with your weight, one of the most overlooked culprits, you are not alone. Weight gain or the inability to lose weight can often create poor sleep habits. Several factors contribute to a fluctuation in weight when it comes to losing sleep. Each of these factors not only makes it more difficult to maintain a healthy weight, they cause us to be at higher risk of heart disease, cardiovascular disease, and further sleep disorders.

Appetite

Sleep causes changes in two specific hunger hormones. The first, ghrelin, stimulates appetite. The second, leptin, is the hormone responsible for suppressing appetite and makes us feel satiety. Those who get less than five hours of sleep have higher levels of ghrelin and significantly lower levels of leptin (Smith, 2018). Not only do you just feel more hunger, you tend to overeat because your hunger hormones are much higher than they normally should be. On top of this, losing sleep inhibits leptin production. Without the adequate levels of leptin, we simply do not get the signal from our brain that we are full, so we continue to eat more.

Additionally, sleep deprivation can trigger a hyper-sensitivity to food stimuli because the brain activities a reward response to food. We crave specific foods like high-calorie and high-sugar foods and are unable to resist the urge to consume more than we should or need to. Even more, our decision-making skills are impaired, so we do not have the right mental capacity to make healthier food choices when we are feeling tired. This affects our metabolic rate.

Diabetes

Sleep impacts blood glucose levels and insulin levels. When you do not sleep enough, your glucose levels rise, triggering insulin to be released and result in frequent fluctuation, even while you sleep. Insulin is how the sugar in our blood gets carried to the muscles and other cells in our body for necessary energy.

When we lose sleep regularly, we tend to crave more carbohydrates or as our body tells us, sweets. This causes further dysregulation without sugar levels and insulin production. Over time, this can result in diabetes, a condition where the body is unable to produce enough insulin or the muscles and cells in the body are unable to absorb the insulin produced. This results in excess glucose to be stored as fat. Since the body does not use up stored fat at a faster rate than more is being added, we gain more weight.

. . .

AGING AND LONGEVITY

Despite advancements in the medical field that can help treat and cure a wide range of illnesses to extend life-expectancy, lack of sleep deteriorates health. Improving sleep is necessary to maintain a healthy life.

Cells Age Quickly

There is no avoiding the aging process, but there are many ways we can slow down the process so that we remain healthy, look, and feel better. When we sleep, we give the cells in our body sufficient time for new cells to grow and replace damaged or abnormal cells.

As we grow older, just one night of poor sleep can cause the cells in our body to age faster. While this will cause more wrinkles and fine lines to show up, it also increases our risk of various diseases like cancer and heart disease.

Life Expectancy

Not getting the recommended hours of sleep each night increases your risk of developing a wide range of medical conditions. When one is at higher risk for multiple health conditions, life expectancy is significantly reduced. Most conditions like obesity, diabetes, cardiovascular disease, and a weakened immune system contribute to the development of other conditions. For instance, if you are considered obese you are at a much greater risk of cardiovascular disease; a weakened immune system puts you at greater risk of developing autoimmune diseases like diabetes. Each of these serious conditions can set off a domino effect for another to occur.

Getting less than five hours of sleep a night has been shown to increase an individual's mortality rate by almost 15% (Rogers, 2008). Sleep is a crucial component that impacts our long-term health and also our day-to-day lives.

CHAPTER 2 - THE BODY'S INTERNAL CLOCK

Understanding your natural internal clock allows you to work with your body's natural rhythm to get a longer and more satisfying night's sleep. Most people struggle with sleep because their body's natural rhythms are out of alignment. When we work to sync these processes, we can improve our sleep; this also can improve our cognitive function. In this chapter, you will not only learn about the rhythms that make the biggest impact on sleep but how our dreams give us a clue about the quality of sleep we are getting.

THE CIRCADIAN RHYTHM

Our circadian rhythm is our internal biological clock.

It cycles through various stages over 24 hours. It is what guides most of our internal processes and regulates our energy levels (Suni, 2020). The body has several circadian rhythms. Some regulate hormone distribution, body temperature regulation, and digestion; other rhythms focus on wakefulness and being alert.

Our circadian rhythm is influenced by our internal processes. The brain sends signals throughout the body to trigger most ebb and flows of each rhythm. These signals, however, can also be impacted by environmental cues, like light, to begin specific body functions and processes. These external cues sync with our brain processes to allow for the right triggers and signals to be sent to the rest of the body, like becoming active or slowing down.

Why Is It Important?

When our circadian rhythm is properly synchronized, we can optimize various functions of the body over the course of 24 hours. Learning to work with your circadian rhythm increases productivity. It is how a majority of the most successful people learn to work more efficiently. There are specific hours in the day when we focus and concentrate easily. Our energy levels fluctuate throughout the day, giving us pockets of time to slow down and re-energize (Suni, 2020).

The circadian rhythm is also what helps us time our meals. It triggers the digestive system to begin breaking down foods and the endocrine system to produce specific hormones that increase energy levels.

It does not remain fixed: our circadian rhythm changes as we get older (Suni, 2020). Our lifestyle and daily habits can also cause a shift in our circadian rhythms. With this understanding, we know that when poor sleep is due to an out of sync rhythm, we can take the necessary steps to return it to its natural cycles.

Most Well-Known Circadian Rhythm

While many rhythms occur in the body, none is more studied and known than the sleep-wake cycle. This cycle also includes our sleep stages that occur in the evening and our energy levels during the day.

The Sleep Cycle

The sleep-wake cycle is one of the most important and well-known circadian rhythms. Our circadian rhythm is naturally in sync with the day and night hours. During the day, our internal clock activates the system necessary to help us stay awake and alert. When the evening hours come out, the clock signals the production of melatonin and initiates processes that help us stay asleep through the night (Suni, 2020). When our rhythm is in proper order, we go through our cycle of restorative sleep which enables us to have enough energy to power through our daytime activities.

Impact on the Circadian Rhythm

How much sleep we get directly impacts the body's other circadian rhythms. When the sleep cycle is disrupted, we unintentionally activate certain systems when they need to remain at rest. For instance, if we frequently wake in the evening and expose ourselves to light, the body stops producing melatonin: this causes us to become alert when we should still be resting.

Fragmented sleep cycles over time can cause us to develop more serious sleep disorders like insomnia, sleep apnea, and excessive daytime sleeping; these will only further contribute to an unhealthy circadian rhythm (NIH, 2013).

To keep our circadian rhythms in sync or to fix an out of balance rhythm, there are a few steps you can take. First, as soon as you wake in the morning, expose yourself to natural sunlight. This simple act can strengthen your circadian rhythm and help correct negative effects from not getting proper sleep during the night. Get yourself on a structured schedule. Your entire day does not have to be planned out; however, you do need to ensure that you are going to bed and waking up at the same time every day, even if you are on vacation or it is the weekend (Suni, 2020).

Increased physical activity, limiting caffeine consumptions, and dimming the lights before bed are additional ways you can realign your circadian rhythm with little effort.

Dream, Dream, Dream

Dreams occur at any stage of the sleep cycle, though the only time we recall our dreams is when they transpire during REM sleep. These dreams are more vivid and can also be confusing and nonsensical. Dreaming that happens during non-REM sleep usually involves more thorough thoughts and reality-based content as they can be pinpointed to actual events or specific times. For most individuals, REM dreaming manifests during the latter part of the sleep period, often during the hours leading up to our waking time.

We typically should spend two hours of our sleep in a dream state. Not recalling dreams is due to not entering the final REM sleep stage in our last sleep cycle or being woken up in the middle of non-REM sleep.

Why We Dream

There are many theories as to why we dream. One is that dreaming is a state in which we store memories from the day and organize all the information gathered from the day. This is especially true when we are working through challenging thoughts and feelings.

It is also suggested that dreaming is a time for the brain to clear away useless information. Through this cleaning process, recent occurrences are replayed and thoroughly analyzed. This can account for why we feel more clarity surrounding certain situations or wake up feeling more confident with recent decisions made.

Though there is debate about the true reason we dream, much research has been conducted. Even if dreaming is just a by-product of sleep that has little purpose, most people will agree that dreams can hold subliminal messages.

Creative and Innovative Ideas

Dreaming has also been linked to increased creativity. During non-REM sleep our memories are strengthened; during REM sleep we fuse our memories more concretely. This results in finding commonalities in problems we are trying to solve as well as a shift in mindset that sees solutions to problems. It can also bring a higher awareness to ourselves and the world around us, which sparks creative thinking.

Ideas that were first just a dream:

- The periodic table
- The song "Yesterday"
- Modern rationalism/analytical geometry
- The character Frankenstein

Many other creative ideas have been sparked by dreams that individuals have had. But, it is not just the dreams that allow us to increase our creativity: it is being able to wake up refreshed and with a clear mind to better look at the problem we are facing and find innovative solutions.

Just Sleep on It

There is a reason why you should wait 24 hours to make a big decision. When we allow ourselves to sleep on finding a solution or making life-changing decisions, we give ourselves time to see things from different points of view. Our subconscious helps us clarify details while we dream.

Entering into a dream state is a natural form of therapy. REM sleep allows us to process emotional trauma experienced through the day or in the past. It provides us with a release from tension, stress, and pent-up emotions (National Sleep Foundation, n.d.). When you experience a good night's sleep after a stressful or emotionally charged day, we feel more clear headed. During REM sleep, we can process our anxiety in a safe and calm state. This is because of noradrenaline, an anxiety molecule that is not produced while we sleep. This provides us with the perfect time to recall emotional, intense memories without suffering from the anxiety effects of doing so (National Sleep Foundation, n.d.).

CHAPTER 3 - SLEEP DEBT

Just as you accumulate debt, when you spend more money than you make, you do the same when you deprive yourself of the right amount of sleep. Sleep debt accumulates over time. When we do not get the sleep our body needs each night, the sleep you lose is added to our debt. In just a short timeframe this debt can become substantial. In the long-term, this will contribute to health conditions.

What Keeps You Up?

There are many reasons why you may struggle with sleep. There are activities that you may be performing late in the day that can make it harder to fall asleep. Additionally, undetected medical conditions can impact your sleep without you even realizing it.

Electronics

The effect of blue light on the brain makes it harder to fall asleep. This is because the light stops melatonin production and triggers brain activity. Remember, our wake-sleep cycle is greatly affected by light, even when it is not sunlight. The light from electronics signals to the brain that we should be alert, so melatonin production is halted. Aside from the light, the visual stimulation keeps our thoughts running on high (National Sleep Foundation, 2020). Even if you use special screen protectors or wear glasses to suppress the blue light that enters the eyes, your brain is still operating on high alert. Our brain activity remains engaged whether we are checking in on social media or enjoying a late-night movie.

Nightcaps

A glass of wine may seem harmless; for many, it can help you fall asleep and stay asleep through the night. Over time, however, we build up a tolerance, and we begin to struggle even more to fall asleep, becoming more dependent on it during the day. There are many ways alcohol can impair whether you drink occasionally or regularly. Consuming alcohol after 3:00 pm will reduce the time you spend in REM sleep. Since alcohol is a sedative, you may find that you fall into a deep sleep rather quickly, but this only throws the rest of your sleep off-balance. You will find that you experience more sleep disturbances as the night goes on, so your quality and quantity of sleep is significantly decreased.

Medical Conditions

Medications make it harder to sleep. Certain conditions like chronic pain or arthritis will cause one to have more fragmented sleep. Mental conditions like anxiety or depression can cause trouble with falling asleep. Cardiovascular and respiratory conditions can impact our sleep cycles causing us to skip deep, restorative sleep. When it comes to understanding our struggles with sleep, we need to carefully examine our overall health. While many sleep problems can be linked to external factors, many more can be the result of an undiagnosed condition. Since poor sleep can also contribute to a developing condition, it is highly recommended that you speak to your doctor—if you have not done so already—about your sleep concerns.

Anxiety, Stress, and Depression

Anxiety, stress, and depression are often conditions that go hand in hand. When you have one of these conditions, it does not take long for another to appear and cause turmoil in your life. The worst is that each of these conditions can make one of the others more severe.

Anxiety and stress are normal experiences of our daily lives. Feeling a little worried, anxious, or fearful about things is normal. It is when these feelings begin to impact our ability to live life normally on our terms that they can become a problem. Both stress and anxiety can make it hard for us to fall asleep. Troubling thoughts of things that have occurred in the past or about things that have yet to happen in the future will keep our thoughts running at high speed as we lay down to sleep. In fact, when we are laying down and not doing anything else except trying to sleep, our thoughts seem to become louder and more distracting. Depression—whether on its own or as a side effect of extreme stress and anxiety—causes many sleep disturbances throughout the night (National Sleep Foundation, 2021).

Learning how to lower our stress, keep anxiety in check, and include activities in our day that allow us to feel valued are key to getting a good night's sleep. We will cover a number of activities to help combat these three conditions so you can sleep better and properly address the root cause of what keeps you from sleeping.

· · ·

SLEEP DEPRIVATION

Skipping a few hours of sleep every once in a while is often unavoidable. Unfortunately, it has also become normal to get well under the eight hours of recommended sleep each night. It is not just adults not prioritizing sleep. School-aged children and teens rarely get the recommended 8 to 10 hours of sleep they need. Regularly getting less sleep than needed leads to sleep deprivation.

Sleep deprivation occurs when we have poor sleeping habits, disruption to our circadian rhythms, a sleep disorder, or medical condition that leads us to not get enough sleep. It can be the absence of sleep completely, partial (where we lose sleep either in the early or late stage of sleep), or selective (we skip specific stages of sleep). If getting less than seven hours of sleep a night is normal for you, it is likely that you are sleep deprived. Even if you may not feel exhausted during the day, sleep deprivation takes a toll on our mental and physical health over time. In the short-term, cognition becomes impaired and our reaction time to external stimuli is slowed down (Committee on Sleep Medicine and Research, n.d.).

Early experimentation on sleep deprivation among animals have shown sleep deprivation to be fatal. This is evident in the Russian and Italian sleep experiments done on dogs, and experiments done on rats in the 1980s and 1990s (Green, 2020). In humans, there have been some studies conducted that prove that severe mental impairments occur when we go days without sleep. Hallucinations, serious mood swings, and paranoia are also present when we try to stay awake for days at a time. The extremely negative effects of sleep deprivation have halted most experimentation to uncover the side effects of this condition. Even the *The Guinness Book of Records* removed the category of individual to stay away from for the most days in a row because of the negative effect (Green, 2020).

Severe sleep deprivation causes individuals to experience microsleeps. These are short periods during waking hours where we fall asleep; most of the time we are completely unaware of these happening. Our body has evolved over the years to create this safeguard against sleep deprivation. We force ourselves to fall asleep when we are sleep deprived. With this evolutionary fail safe imposed we are less likely to die from direct effects of sleep deprivation. However, the negative impacts it has on our cognitive function, alertness, and reflexes can cause fatal accidents (Committee on Sleep Medicine and Research, n.d.).

. . .

Do You Have a Deficit?

If you consistently get fewer hours of sleep then what your body needs, that is a sleep deficit. Most individuals need between 6-10 hours of sleep, with the average consensus being eight hours. The average person tends to only get about six hours of sleep a day, and many of those individuals are adding close to four hours of sleep debt every night if they require 10 hours of sleep. In just a week, they are only averaging 42 hours of sleep when they should be getting closer to 70. This is the same as though they stayed up for three days straight: in two weeks their total hours of sleep loss is equivalent to staying awake for one week straight. That is quite a lot of sleep to be missing out on.

Signs You May Have A Sleep Deficit

There are many things that can cause you to lose out on the sleep you need. While it may seem like staying up an extra half hour to finish a show or staying out an hour longer to catch up with friends seems harmless, even the littlest bit of sleep that you lose can quickly add up. There are some red flags you want to be aware of when it comes to building up a sleep debt.

1. A high sleep debt does not always give you

clear signs. You may not feel tired at all after sleeping for only a few hours for long periods of time. This does not mean that your body is not giving you red flags that you are in fact in need of serious sleep. We may not feel tired as a result of not getting enough sleep, physically and mentally; however, we will notice a decline in performance.

2. Brain fog is another indication that you are accumulating too much sleep debt. Brain fog happens when you have difficulty recalling basic information that you should know without having to think about it, like your phone number, child's birthday, or what you just walked into the kitchen for. Brian fog is often brushed off and laughable, but it can be a red flag that you are in need of sleep.

3. Having trouble with your vision is another indication of a sleep deficit.

4. You will also not have more trouble remembering things: did you lose track of where you set your phone down or where you placed the car keys? Ever put on a pot of water to make tea and honey when you smell something burning? Do you remember that is what you intended to do? There are many absent indeed occurrences and forgetful

       episodes that are actually clues you are not getting enough sleep.

5. Dozing off during the day is a clear sign that you are in serious debt with your sleep. Drowsiness during the day, to the point where you drift off even for short periods of time, is a sign you need to catch up on your sleep debt.

6. Long-term signs you may be suffering from a serious sleep debt is weight gain or difficulty losing weight. Since sleep is vital for maintaining a healthy weight. When we begin to skip too much of it, our body will begin to put on extra pounds.

Never lose hope: you can always pay off your sleep debt. Even if you struggle now to get to sleep or stay asleep there are ways to repay your debt. It will not, however, happen by trying to catch up on your sleep in one night. You will need to add an additional hour or two to your sleep schedule to help deplete your deficit. Those who are chronically sleep deprived may need a few months to get their body into its natural sleep/wake cycle.

The best approach to eliminate a sleep debt is a slow and steady pace. Trying to bump up your bedtime by a few hours on the first night will only lead to tossing and turning. Instead, move up your bedtime by just 15 minutes at a time (National Sleep Foundation, n.d.). This lets your internal clock gradually shift and get used to its new routine.

You can also assist your natural clock by letting it take the reins for a while. When you are feeling tired in the evening, go to bed. Do not try to force yourself to stay up an extra hour or two until your usual bedtime. If you do not need to be up at a specific time, avoid setting an alarm, and allow your body to wake up on its own. The first few days you do this you may find that you sleep for 10 hours without a problem, but may still feel slightly lethargic during the day. As you continue to trust your body's natural system, you will find that you are sleeping for fewer hours while feeling more rejuvenated and energized the next day. You will begin to notice a sleep pattern emerge that is specific for your body. You can track how many hours you tend to sleep naturally; this will be the hours your body needs to be in its sleep state for maximum restorative benefits. Now you will be able to tell when you are getting the sleep you need and when you are building up a debt. Knowing this information will help you avoid a substantial sleep debt that seriously impacts your daily functionality.

· · ·

WHAT ABOUT OVERSLEEPING?

Oversleeping in the mornings or on the weekends may just be a result of trying to catch up on a sleep debt. Sleeping in, however, will only make falling asleep in the evening more difficult and has the opposite effects on reducing your sleep debt. While you may get a few extra hours of sleep in the morning, this can result in restlessness and losing hours of sleep during the night.

Daytime sleep may help you get the hours of sleep you need, but feeling fatigued and sleeping too much during daylight hours is not ideal. Oversleeping during the daylight hours can be caused by many factors. If you are severely sleep deprived, it is understandable that you would sleep more during the day. This can, however, be a red flag that there are more concerning healthy issues causing your extreme tiredness (National Sleep Foundation, 2021).

Even if you are not actually sleeping during the day, feeling drowsy or physically fatigued for most of the day can be a serious issue as well. When we are feeling this lethargic during the day it impairs our motor abilities, putting us at greater risk of accidents. It also interferes with our daily activities and performance levels.

If you find yourself dozing off during the day when

you should not be, this is a clear indication that you are suffering from excessive daytime sleepiness. Individuals who drift off while watching television, sitting inactive in public places (like during a meeting or at the theatres), while riding in a car without stops for at least an hour, or even when they have stopped at a red light while driving all point to sleep struggles (National Sleep Foundation, 2021).

CHAPTER 4 - QUALITY VS. QUANTITY SLEEP

Getting the right amount of sleep is important, but it will not matter how many hours you sleep if you simply do not get quality sleep. Quality sleep means you are spending enough time in each of the sleep stages. When we are not getting enough REM sleep our brain function is impaired. When our deep non-REM stages are interrupted we will still feel tired. Too much light sleep makes it easier for us to be woken up from sleep and will make it harder to fall back asleep. The quality of your sleep can have a bigger impact on health and happiness. This is just as important for children as it is for adults (Leavitt, 2019).

.

. . .

OPTIMAL SLEEP

To get the full restorative benefits from sleeping you need to get the right number of hours of sleep as well as quality sleep. This means you are going through the sleep stages the proper number of times. For one to decrease their sleep debt they need to focus on both the hours of sleep they get as well as the quality of that sleep. We need to be spending more time in a restorative, deep sleep.

What Is Proper Sleep?

While the total number of hours needed for proper sleep will vary from one person to another, it is ideal to aim for eight hours of sleep every night. You may need slightly more or you may need slightly less. Only when you get into a consistent sleeping routine will you be able to judge if you are getting adequate sleep or not. About 25% of our sleeping time is spent in REM sleep, another 25% is spent in deep restorative sleep, and the remaining 50% is spent in light sleep or the first two stages of non-REM sleep. As we get older the time spent in deep sleep declines as we need less of it (Leavitt, 2019).

You should be able to fall asleep in 30 minutes or less. If it takes you longer than this to fall asleep you are fighting with your natural rhythm or you may suffer from a sleep disorder. If you find that you are tossing, turning, and trying to force yourself to sleep, you are better off getting up (LeWine, 2014). Pick up a book to read, do some light stretches, write out your thoughts, and try again in 20 minutes. Sometimes you just need to get up for a bit and go to another room to reset. Resist the urge to turn on the television or scroll social media. You want to encourage the mind and body to wind down, not revert it back up (LeWine, 2014).

Proper sleep also means you are sleeping throughout the night. If you wake up in the middle of the night for more than three nights a week then you are not getting proper sleep.

Proper Sleep for Children

Sleep recommendations for children have changed over the years. As new research is conducted it is becoming more evident that children need more sleep for proper development and learning. If children are not sleeping properly, parents will also lose sleep. If parents have poor sleeping habits, their children will often develop poor sleeping habits as well. This results in a cycle of both parents and children contributing to other others sleeping issues. To break the cycle we need to first, as parents, ensure we have proper sleep habits established. Then we need to understand how our children's sleep changes over time to help them adapt to right sleep patterns (National Sleep Foundation, n.d.).

Recommended Sleep By Age

Newborns from 0 to 3 months should get 15-18 hours of sleep. Newborns should not get less than 11 hours of sleep and no more than 19 hours of sleep.

Infants from 4 to 11 months should get 13-16 hours of sleep. Infants should not get less than 10 hours of sleep and no more than 18 hours of sleep.

Toddlers from 1 to 5 years of age should be getting 11-14 hours of sleep. Toddlers should not get less than nine hours of sleep and should not get more than 16 hours of sleep.

School-aged children from 6 to 13 should get 9-11 hours of sleep. School-aged children should not sleep for less than seven hours or for more than 12 hours.

Teenagers from the age of 14 to 17 should get 8-10 hours of sleep. Teenagers should not get less than seven hours of sleep and no more than 11 hours of sleep.

These age recommendations are based on a wide range of research and in-depth studies. Each recommendation also states that the number of hours a child has for sleep should never go under or over at any time. While children's sleep patterns can be erratic, it is best to teach them proper sleep habits while they are young than to have them struggle with sleep conditions when they are older (National Sleep Foundation, 2015).

Sleep Regressions

Sleep regressions are a natural part of growing up for your child. You may have a perfectly sleeping child and suddenly you and your little one have multiple sleepless nights. If your child is fighting to get to sleep in the evening or is having more frequent wakings throughout the night, they are in a sleep regression. While sleep regressions may feel like they suddenly spring up out of nowhere, they typically occur around the same similar milestone in most children (de Bellefonds, 2020).

The most common sleep regression occurs around 4, 6, 8, 12, and 18 months as well as around their second birthday. Some children will not experience each regression: others may struggle long with regression, though most last for a few weeks.

When sleep regressions do occur, it is important to continue with your already established sleep routines. Continue to go through your evening routine with your child. Most parents find that sleep regressions occur when their child is sleeping too much during the day which is having a negative impact on their evening sleep. This is often the time where naps will either be cut from their day or shortened.

Sleep regression also coincided with big developmental milestones. Babies who are just learning to move around, walk, and jump may have more resistance to sleeping, so they can practice their new mobility skills. Babies who learn to talk may stay up longer babbling or want to hear your voice a little longer to learn new sounds. Additionally, growth spurts, brain development, and bigger life changes (like moving or going on vacation) can also contribute to sleep regressions.

Getting Kids on a Sleep Schedule

Newborns do not yet have a clearly defined circadian rhythm. It is not until they are at least three months that they begin to develop a sleep/wake cycle. Until this point babies are encouraged to sleep most of their days and nights. After the 3-month milestone, they begin to settle into a more structured sleep routine, which we continue to change every few months when naps are shortened and eliminated.

Even though sleep patterns will change, parents are encouraged to begin practicing proper sleep hygiene routines with their newborns and infants. It is important to create a calming bedtime routine that will help your child grow into the habit of getting ready for bed. Reading, bathtime, and a small healthy snack can all be included in a bedtime routine. As your child gets older their bedtime routine will also change. You may rock your newborn to sleep, but at around 6 months, this rocking may stop and be replaced with singing a lullaby as they lay in their bed or read them a story (de Bellefonds, 2020).

It is important that sleep routines are practiced every night, even while vacationing or visiting family members. It is also important that when sleep regression occurs you do not revert back to old habits you used to try to get your baby to sleep quickly. Newborns will wake frequently in the evening because they need to be fed or changed; between 6 and 9 months of age however, nighttime feeding should not be occurring as frequently. When the 8-month sleep regression happens, you do not want to go back to feeding your baby just to get him back to sleep.

You want to teach your child effective skills to soothe themselves back to sleep. Utilizing old tricks will only prolong the sleepless nights.

• • •

IMPROVING SLEEP IN CHILDREN

Much of the things you will learn to help improve your own sleep are the same ways you can help improve your child's sleep.

1. Have a clear bedtime routine.
2. Stick with consistent going to bed and wake-up times.
3. Perform relaxing activities before bed.
4. Avoid drinking water at least an hour before bed.
5. Dim the lights, use a sound machine, and check the room temperature.
6. Ensure your child has a safe space to sleep in.
7. Do not let your child watch scary shows or cartoons before bed.

CHAPTER 5 - INSOMNIA

Falling asleep and staying asleep are red flags of insomnia. When we ignore these signs we can suffer from significant sleep deficits. Insomnia is a common sleep disorder that can disrupt sleep at least once a week; those with chronic insomnia will suffer for at least three nights of poor sleep a week. Nearly 60% of adults are diagnosed with insomnia, and even more go undiagnosed (Bhaskar et al, 2016).

SLEEP-ONSET INSOMNIA

Sleep-onset insomnia is when you have trouble falling asleep. You may be ready to sleep and even feel exhausted but as soon as you lay down you begin to toss and turn. This type of insomnia makes itself known most often during your daytime hours. You will notice you are more irritable, fatigued, and unable to concentrate. What causes this condition to be worse is the simple fact that your inability to fall asleep, despite how tired you are, becomes frustrated. Your anger for not being able to fall asleep causes you to struggle even more with getting to sleep. By the time you finally do sleep, the total hours you can spend sleeping is significantly cut short (National Sleep Foundation, 2020).

Onset insomnia is often the result of psychological or psychiatric issues. Stress, anxiety, and depression are the most common factors that led to onset insomnia. Individuals who have another sleep disorder are also more likely to develop onset insomnia. Lifestyle changes can also contribute to onset insomnia as well as environmental factors like a noisy location and electronics (National Sleep Foundation, 2020).

Caffeine and stimulants will worsen this type of insomnia. Short-term life stressors will also make insomnia worse because they make the psychological factors harder, like anxiety and depression.

Sleep Maintenance Insomnia

If you have trouble staying asleep or find that you are

waking up too early and unable to fall back asleep once you wake, you may suffer from sleep maintenance insomnia. This type of insomnia takes away from your hours of sleep in two ways. First, by waking up frequently you are not getting the quality or length of sleep you need. Second, when you are unable to fall back asleep, you begin to worry and stress about not getting enough sleep; this makes it more difficult to fall asleep again. Many people find themselves in a situation where it is still too early for them to be awake, but at the same time, is too late for them to try to get back to sleep. Since we tend to move into lighter sleep as the night progresses, it is easier for one to be stirred awake. This is why many struggle to get back to sleep when they wake (National Sleep Foundation, 2020).

Like onset insomnia, maintenance income can be linked to some psychological issues like depression. More often, though, it is associated with another medical condition like reflux disease, sleep apnea, and restless leg syndrome. Women are more likely to suffer from this type of insomnia than their male counterparts (National Sleep Foundation, 2020).

Hybrid Insomnia

Hybrid insomnia is the combination of being unable

to fall asleep and stay asleep, many also specifically struggle with waking up too early. Hybrid insomnia can also refer to those who shift between onset insomnia and maintenance insomnia. For a few weeks, you may struggle to fall asleep, or for a few weeks, you may struggle with staying asleep. You don't necessarily have to suffer from both forms of insomnia at the same time but do struggle with both (National Sleep Foundation, 2020).

MISCONCEPTION ABOUT INSOMNIA

1. Even if you only suffer from acute insomnia —meaning at least once a week you are not getting the sleep you need—there are short and long-term effects. Your productivity will suffer in work or school life. You also are at a greater risk of mental and physical health conditions including depression, heart disease, and obesity.
2. Insomnia can be addressed a number of ways. Many find they are able to correct their sleep struggles with a change in their sleep schedule and making minor lifestyle changes. Others may require additional help to confront the underlying issue that contributes to their sleepless nights.

3. Insomnia is more than just your thoughts running wild. Many believe that they struggle to sleep because it is all in their heads. While your thoughts do have a major rule in your inability to fall asleep most of the time, there are many other factors that contribute to insomnia that have nothing to do with the thoughts that are making you worry or stress.

4. You may be getting enough sleep but still feel tired, and insomnia is not the culprit. Most of us rely on alarm clocks to wake us up when we need to be up. If your alarm gets off while you are in the middle of REM sleep, you are going to wake up feeling tired and will often feel tired for a good portion of the first half of your day. However, this does not mean you are struggling with sleep or you are getting enough sleep.

5. Napping does not actually help when you have insomnia. Since most people would only be able to nap in the later hours of the day, this can actually make your insomnia worse. While you will be getting in a few extra hours of sleep, it will make your evening sleep regime just as stressful and difficult.

Children can also suffer from insomnia and is referred to as behavioral insomnia in childhood. This type of childhood in children is more specifically focused on the struggles to go to sleep. Either they have not learned proper coping skills to fall asleep easily, so they need to be rocked or have gotten used to falling asleep while watching television. They may also put off going to sleep by requesting additional items to "help" them sleep like an extra glass of water, another story, or to use the restroom again. Children may also utilize a combination of these two strategies to avoid going to sleep (Pacheco, 2020).

CHAPTER 6 - SLEEP DISTURBANCES

Sleep disturbances make it difficult to get quality sleep, some of these may occur once in a while, but even less frequent sleep disturbances can have adverse effects over time. While most sleep disturbances can be attributed to external factors, there are a few that you may be unaware of. In this chapter, you learn some of the most common and some not some common conditions that cause disruption to sleep.

Sleepwalking and Night Terrors

Sleepwalking and night terrors are not huge thieves of sleep, but they can make sleeping unpleasant. Both these occurrences can interfere with the quality of sleep as they often take you out of a restorative sleep. Though it is more common in younger children and teens, it also interferes with parental sleep.

Sleepwalking

Sleepwalking mimics how someone would walk around as if they were awake. Sleepwalking is the act of getting up and walking around while you are sound asleep. Your eyes are often open while this is occurring, but they will have a more glazed over or glossy expression. The person who is sleepwalking is unaware of what is really going on in their surroundings. They will not respond to others when they speak to them and often do not take notice of anything moving around them. This is more likely to happen in the earlier hours of sleep, usually an hour or two after you have fallen asleep. These episodes can last up to 30 minutes. It is difficult to wake someone who is in the middle of a sleepwalking episode. When the person is woken, they are disoriented and in a state of confusion (Suni, 2020).

Night Terrors

Nightmares and night terrors are commonly confused with one another. Nightmares are unpleasant dreams and are common in both children and adults. These dreams are vivid and often start off as any normal dream but become more terrifying the longer you are in the dream state. When you are experiencing a nightmare you will often feel threatened, you sweat, your heart rate increases, and you tend to wake up and remember many details or at least know that you have had one.

Night terrors are less common than nightmares. They are more prevalent in children under the age of 13. Adults can, however, suffer from night terrors. Night terrors, unlike nightmares, occur when you are in non-REM sleep and in the deepest stage of sleep. Like sleepwalking, they tend to happen an hour or two after falling asleep. These episodes last 10 to 20 minutes; when they have subsided, the person will often not wake fully, but instead, drift back to their deep sleep state (National Sleep Foundation, 2020).

Night terrors involve screaming episodes, feelings of intense fear, and erratic thrashing about. They are generally not remembered by those who experience them. It is also quite calming for one to experience night terrors and sleepwalking at the same time.

Because night terrors are not usually remembered, they are often more terrifying for someone who witnesses the event. When you are having a night terror your eyes may be wide open, given off the appearance that you are awake when you are not. You are inconsolable: attempting to comfort you or wake you will result in more thrashing and erratic reactions.

Night terrors are experienced by those who have an anxiety disorder. They can be triggered by stress, illnesses, and changes in sleep schedules. Those that suffer from restless leg syndrome, sleep apnea, and sleep deprivation are more likely to experience night terrors (National Sleep Foundation, 2020).

What Can You Do About Them?

Sleepwalking and night terrors tend to run in families, which can make it easier to identify if you are experiencing them. Those who suffer from frequent night terrors or sleepwalking episodes should take extra measures to ensure they are getting the right amount of sleep each night. You should also take extra safety precautions to ensure that when an episode does occur you will not injure yourself or others.

Alcohol is also believed to initiate night terrors and sleepwalking. Cutting back or completely eliminating alcohol from your diet can help decrease the frequency of these disturbances.

Incorporate stress reduction activities throughout your day, not just before you go to bed. Light reading, meditating, and listening to calming music before bed can help you feel more relaxed and get you in the mood for sleep. This, however, is not enough to combat all the stress that has accumulated during the day. Making time for additional meditation sessions, yoga, walking in nature, and taking time to sit quietly to decompress is essential (Suni, 2020).

Nocturnal Lagophthalmos

Nocturnal lagophthalmos is a condition where one sleeps with the eyes open. Closing the eyes during the day is not an issue, but when you sleep the nerves or muscles prevent the eyes from closing. This is typically the result of nerve or muscle damage in the face or behind the eyes. Stroke, blunt force trauma to the face, cranial damage of the seventh nerve, autoimmune conditions, and tumors are some of the most common causes for this condition. Damage to the eyelids can also lead to nocturnal lagophthalmos.

How Does This Impact Sleep?

While this condition is not life-threatening it can increase the risk of further eye problems. Severe dry eyes or even damage to the eye can occur. Additionally, when the eyes remain open while you sleep, it exposes you to external light which can cause you to wake up before you are ready.

There are options to help treat this condition, both surgical and nonsurgical treatments. Depending on the root causes and severity there are several surgeries that can be considered. Non-surgical options include using artificial tears, keeping a humidifier running while you sleep, using surgical tape to help keep the eyelids closed as you sleep, and wearing a type of sleep goggles to help protect the eyes (Cafasso, 2018).

Restless Leg Syndrome (RLS)

Restless leg syndrome frequently occurs in the evening hours, but the symptoms can occur whenever you are sitting still or just resting briefly. This condition causes the uncontrollable desire to move the legs. You will usually experience an uncomfortable sensation; despite how much you move around to alleviate the discomfort, you only find temporary relief from it.

There is no known direct cause for this condition, but those who have lower levels of iron in the brain or have a family history of RLS are more likely to suffer from it. Restless leg syndrome causes an indescribable sensation in the lower limbs. Some feel a throbbing discomfort, crawling sensation, or pulling of the muscles. While the sensation may vary from one person to another, the nagging urge to relieve the discomfort remains constant from each diagnosis (Mayo Clinic, 2020).

This condition can severely impact the length and quality of sleep. Those who suffer from RLS often note that the uncomfortable sensation worsens as the night goes on, this can make staying asleep impossible, if they manage to get to sleep at all.

What Can Be Done About It?

If you suffer from RLS there are a few ways that you can help alleviate the sensation keeping you up. Most find that walking or moving the legs will diminish symptoms, but once you stop or sit, the effects return.

Iron supplements can help reduce the side effects of RLS. Lifestyle changes can help those with mild or moderate RLS. These changes include avoiding alcohol, quitting smoking, starting an exercise routine (specifically one that includes leg-stretching moves), leg massages, warm baths, heating pads or ice packs, and making adjustments to your sleep patterns. There are prescription medications that might help with more severe RLS diagnosis, but most of these medications are not designed to treat RLS specifically.

Most medications are used to treat seizures or Parkinson's disease. Though they have been shown to be effective for RLS, they are options you will want to carefully consider or only use as a last resort (Mayo Clinic, 2020).

Sleep Apnea

Sleep apnea is a condition in which breathing momentarily stops during your sleeping hours. The muscles of the lungs and respiratory tract briefly stop moving. Most individuals are unaware when this occurs because it happens for such a short time. Even so, brief pauses in breathing will interfere with sleep. Over time, the condition can worsen. Not all sleep apnea is the same.

Those who suffer from sleep apnea are more likely to be obese and are at greater risk for cardiovascular disease. They are also more likely to be in automobile accidents and fall asleep while driving (The Lung Association, 2020).

There are three common types of sleep apnea (The Lung Association, 2020):

Obstructive (OSA): If you suffer from excessive daytime sleepiness the most common cause is obstructive sleep apnea. OSA occurs when there is a blockage in the upper airways making it difficult for air to pass through causing a reduction in airflow. This typically occurs five or more times in an hour which contributes to repetitive snoring; repetitive snoring is a common indication that one suffers from obstructive sleep apnea, but since the snoring occurs while you are asleep it is difficult to know when it is happening.

Central: Central sleep apnea occurs when the brain does not send signals to the muscles necessary for breathing. The airways are not blocked but breathing stops due to faulty messages being sent from the brain.

Mixed: With mixed sleep apnea there are both blocked airways and missed messages from the brain to initiate breathing.

All cases of sleep apnea results in the individuals being woken partially from sleep in order to resume breathing. Sleep becomes fragmented and the quality of sleep is lowered.

Sleep apnea is highly underdiagnosed. The only way to get a definitive diagnosis is to undergo a sleep study, which is an overnight test. Once sleep apnea is confirmed there are several treatments options (Mayo Clinic, 2020).

1. Positive Airway Pressure Devices

The most common way to treat sleep apnea is through the use of a breathing mask. This mask is worn while sleeping to increase air pressure to prevent the airway from becoming clocked. The air mask is connected to a machine by a flexible tube. There are a variety of machines this can be hooked up to, and each adjust air pressure to varying degrees.

2. Oral Appliances

Oral appliances are placed in the mouth and resemble mouth guards. They help keep the lower jaw position slightly forward as you sleep. These appliances are used primarily as a first line of treatment for sleep apnea. They keep the airways open so air can flow freely while you sleep.

3. Hypoglossal Neuro-Stimulation Therapy

Those suffering from obstructive sleep apnea can choose a neuro-stimulation therapy treatment. This utilizes an implant placed inside the body to stimulate and strengthen the muscles used for breathing. It helps individuals control breathing and regulate air pressure in a similar way that positive airway pressure devices do but without having to be hooked up to a face mask throughout the night.

Neuro-stimulation therapy can also be used for those suffering from central sleep apnea. This treatment uses an implant to stimulate the nerves in the chest and to trigger the muscles that control breathing to keep working. The signals sent from the implant act in the same way as the signals from the brain are supposed to act.

4. Weight Loss

More than half of the individuals who suffer from sleep apnea are overweight. Losing weight can help reduce the side effects of sleep apnea, especially those who suffer from snoring. If you are overweight and have been diagnosed with sleep apnea, or if you believe you suffer from this condition, losing weight is the first natural treatment that can be used to combat sleep apnea.

5. Positional Therapy

For many, sleep apnea may only be present when you sleep in a certain position, like on your back. Learning to sleep on your side can eliminate the airway from becoming blocked and significantly reduce the effects of sleep apnea. There are different techniques and products that can be used during sleep to help encourage side sleeping. This type of sleep apnea treatment is better suited for those who have mild sleep apnea. In more severe cases of sleep apnea, the potion you lay in while sleeping could still cause collapsing with the airways.

NARCOLEPSY

Narcolepsy is a sleep disorder that causes excessive daytime sleep. Sleeping too much during the day causes fragmented and poor sleep in the evening. Individuals with this condition have trouble staying awake for long periods of time (Mayo Clinic, 2020). Aside from excessive daytime sleep, those with narcolepsy may also experience:

- Cataplexy (loss of muscle control that is trigger by a strong emotion)
- Hallucinations (dream-like experiences occur while the individual is awake)
- Sleep paralysis (loss of muscle control in the limbs and abdomen)
- Sleep disruptions (often vivid nightmares during late night sleeping)

Those with narcolepsy have unclear sleep wake cycles which makes them fall asleep involuntarily. This condition affects the system in the brain that sends signals to the rest of the body that it needs to remain alert. Mixed signals are being sent out to different parts of the body. For instance, signals from the brainstem activate areas of the body to wake up while signals from the hypothalamus are not being triggered to produce chemicals (hypocretin) that promote this alertness. The inability of the brain to produce hypocretin is what causes individuals to feel more drowsy and unable to remain awake for long (Mayo Clinic, 2020).

What Can Be Done About It?

Unfortunately, there is no cure for narcolepsy, but there are options to help manage the condition. First, understand when you are prone to have sleeping episodes and what triggers them. There will be times where you are more fatigued during the day and activities that can cause you to lose muscle control. What you eat can have a major impact on your symptoms. Daily exercise can also help you feel more energized and alert.

Medications are available to help manage narcolepsy, but they need to be administered at the right times. Tracking your symptoms and when you take your medication is essential for getting on a more consistent routine.

Though you may struggle to stick to a sleep routine, practicing good sleeping habits can have positive effects. Limiting caffeine, incorporating short naps in the day, and sticking to a regular bedtime can improve your condition (Mayo Clinic, 2020).

It is also important to find the right support group. Struggling with narcolepsy can make you feel isolated and misunderstood. Even if close friends and relatives know your diagnosis they will not fully understand how you struggle every day. A support group of individuals who truly understand what you are dealing with can alleviate the isolating effects.

CHAPTER 7 - CREATING A SLEEP SANCTUARY

External factors contribute to a majority of sleep troubles, therefore, we need to first address where you sleep and how to create the right sleeping environment. You may know that certain factors will improve sleep, and you may have taken some of the steps to address these issues. Creating the ideal sleep setting—from mattress to room temperature as well as the smells and colors in your room—can improve sleep dramatically. Be sure to address all the areas of your sleep environment discussed in this chapter.

WHERE DO YOU SLEEP?

Where you sleep will directly impact the quality and quantity of sleep you get. Establishing the right sleeping environment can help alleviate many of the struggles you have with sleep. When we create an environment that promotes a sleep mindset, we will fall asleep faster and stay asleep for longer. Your environment should be inviting and clear of clutter.

Choosing the Right Mattress/Bed

The space of your bedroom will determine the size of mattress you get. The mattress you sleep on should be comfortable and supportive. The right mattress will provide you with the right amount of firmness to alleviate pain and pressure of specific points in the body.

Most mattresses need to be replaced after 10 years, but some will need an upgrade before then. If you find your mattress is sagging, feels lumpy, or it has holes or tears in it, it is time for a new one. There are mattresses specially designed to maximize comfort for all body types. There are also ones designed to accommodate preferred sleeping positions, sleeping next to a partner that tosses and turns, and ones you can adjust the stiffness and temperature of.

When choosing the right mattress you want to take into consideration the type of mattress, firmness, and durability. Mattresses can be made from a wide range of materials, the most popular include foam, inner-spring, latex, or a hybrid. Foam mattresses are ideal for couples and have a higher contouring rate to relieve pressure and isolate motion. Innersprings are budget-friendly but have limited motion isolation and lack support. Latex mattresses offer a higher quality material that is more durable, providing more support than most other mattress types. A hybrid mattress combines two or more types to maximize comfort. Hybrids tend to have a short layer of coil springs topped with a foam or latex system (Sleep-.org, 2020).

The firmness of the mattress will provide the right amount of support for your body type. This takes into consideration your weight and the position you tend to sleep in. Those who are under 130 pounds and tend to sleep on their side will want a much softer mattress. Those who are between 130 and 230 pounds will want a medium to firm mattress. Individuals who are over 230 pounds or who prefer to sleep on their back or stomach will want a firmer mattress.

Durability is also important. You want to get the most years out of your mattress, so choosing the right type and firmness for your body type will impact the longevity of your mattress. It can be a bit of an investment to buy a new mattress, but it is well worth the price. To increase the quality of sleep, your mattress will make all the difference.

The Right Pillow

Pillows do not get as much attention as mattresses do when it comes to improving sleep, but they can be just as important. Pillows allow you to maintain the right sleep posture through the night. It keeps the knees, hips, spine, head, and neck properly aligned for optimal sleep. The right pillow is essential for providing more comfort as you sleep. They specifically relieve tension in the neck by providing the right support for the head.

If you are not sure when the last time you replaced your pillows would be, it is probably time for a new one. If your pillow is worn out, easy to fold, or you need to constantly fluff your pillow throughout the night it is time for a new one. Unlike mattresses, pillows should be replaced frequently, typically every 18 months. Even if you choose a higher quality pillow you will need to replace these at least every two years (Sleep.org, 2020).

When it comes to choosing the right pillow, you have plenty of options. First, consider the fill. Down pillows give you an extra soft area to lay your head. These are typically made from goose or duck feathers or a combination of features and other fillings. A high-quality down pillow will be hypoallergenic and can be more expensive. There are also synthetic down or polyester fills: these will provide a little more firmness to support your head. These pillows are less expensive but flatten more quickly over time and therefore, need to be replaced more often. Wool pillows are great for those with severe allergies as they are resistant to mold and dust mites. These pillows are highly recommended to help regulate body temperature as they absorb excess moisture from the head and neck. These pillows are more firm than others but can last much longer as well. Latex and memory foam pillows are ideal for those that need extra support for their necks and head. These pillows restrict movement while you sleep to keep the body in proper alignment. Latex pillows are also mold and dust mite resistance. Memory foam pillows retain heat: even if they are made with built-in ventilation, they can cause discomfort for those who sweat more (Gniazdowski, 2019).

The next thing to look at when choosing the right pillow is weight. Down pillows and synthetic pillows are lightweight which lets you reshape them and move them with more ease as you sleep. Memory foam and latex have a heavier feel so they retain their shape. Once you have decided on a heavier or lightweight fill you want to choose the best quality. A higher-quality fill will be more expensive but it will also mean you get more life out of your pillow (Gniazdowski, 2019).

Finally, consider the size of your pillow. A standard-size pillow is the go-to choice for most people. A larger pillow may be preferred by some, but keep in mind, your pillow should keep the head, neck, and shoulders in proper alignment to the spine. If you are looking for a specific support pillow these may vary in size as well.

Your sleep position should also be taken into consideration when choosing the right pillow, just as you would for choosing the right mattress. Side sleepers will find more comfort in a firmer pillow that is a little thicker than others. Those who choose to sleep on their stomach will find more comfort in a softer pillow. If you are a back sleeper you might want to consider a softer pillow. If you suffer from neck or back pain and sleep on your back you will want a pillow that is soft but also provide the right support (Gniazdowski, 2019).

Always keep your pillows and cases clean. Pillows can attract dust buildup that interferes with breathing while you sleep.

Bedding

The sheets and blankets you have on your bed can

also affect your sleep. You want to have the right bedding to keep you warm, but the color of that bedding also plays a role in your sleep. Bedding impacts sleep in two ways. First, the comfort of the bedding, how it feels, how it regulates temperature, and how it can help you fall asleep and stay asleep. Second, the look of the bedding can promote a sleep mindset.

Bedding should keep your body temperature within the right zone. During colder months you might want to have an extra blanket or comforter on the bed. During warmer months a simple sheet or light blanket will keep you cool enough to sleep through the night.

Microfiber bedding is ideal for those who tend to feel cold most of the time because they are also easy to care for. Cotton sheets are better for those who feel hotter. When choosing cotton sheets, pay attention to fiber length. Extra long staple fiber results in a softer and more durable sheet. With cotton sheets, thread count has little impact on comfort or quality. Always keep your bedding clean. Just like pillow cases, bedding will easily attract dust and dander. Also, it simply feels better to crawl into a bed with clean sheets on it.

When it comes to colors, warm colors or calming

colors that help you feel relaxed will ease you into sleep. Bedrooms that are painted or prominently display blue, yellow or green tones tend to help individuals drift off to sleep. Purple, brown, and gray tones can make it harder to fall asleep.

External temperature

Room temperature is also important to consider. You may set your thermostat slightly higher before going to bed, but then find yourself waking up too hot in the middle of the night. On the other hand, you may set the room colder before going to bed and wake up freezing. Our body temperature fluctuates as we sleep, so we need to set the right temperature to accommodate these fluctuations without disturbing our sleep.

Setting the Right Temperature

Room temperature needs to suit your natural body temperature. The ideal sleep temperature will depend on your own body temperature. For most, keeping the room around 68 degrees Fahrenheit is ideal. A slightly cooler room can be better for sleep. Experiment with different temperatures if you find yourself waking up too hot or too cold.

Keeping a fan running will help regulate the room

temperature through the night. If possible, open a window to keep temperatures cooler during hot summer months, but only if external noises will not interfere with sleep.

What you wear to bed will also impact your body temperature. Sleepwear should be light and non-restrictive. The more comfortable you are in what you wear to bed the better you will sleep. Many people find that sleeping naked is more comfortable as it keeps the body temperature consistently lower.

Air Circulation

It is important to have proper air circulation and air quality. This not only aids in regulating your breathing as you sleep but is important for your overall health. Proper air circulation will also ensure that dust mites are cleared from the air. This is especially important for those that suffer from allergies. A ceiling fan helps keep air moving around. Air purifiers are also an option. These not only push clean fresh air into the room, they remove particles that can cause breathing troubles. The air that flows from the purifier will typically be cooler so it keeps the room temperature lower.

Humidity Levels

Humidity levels need to be considered when establishing your sleep environment. Not only does humidity impact how comfortable you sleep, but it can also impact how well you breathe as you sleep. You want humidity levels to be between 30% and 50%. High levels will keep your room warm but will also make it difficult for moisture to evaporate from the body. When humidity levels are too high, this increases the risk of mold buildup. Even a small amount of mold can produce spores that make it difficult to sleep and impairs our breathing.

Light

Light is one of the most crucial components of your circadian rhythm. Sleeping in a dark room encourages sleep. Even the smallest amount of light, like that emitted from an alarm clock, can hinder sleep. Making small adjustments to the lighting in your room can improve your evening hours of sleep.

Warm Lighting

Warm and low-colored lights should be used in your bedroom. This will cause the least amount of stimulation in the brain. As discussed earlier, avoid screen time before bed. While it is common to have a television in your bedroom, the blue light from the screen will keep brain activity high. The light from electronics will activate brain waves and disrupt your circadian rhythm (National Sleep Foundation, 2020). If you do have a television in your room, turn it off at least an hour before bedtime. Also avoid using cell phones, computers, or tablets in that hour leading up to bedtime.

If you have an alarm clock near your bed, consider moving it further away from the bed or turning it away from where you sleep so the light is facing away from you. Turning the alarm away also eliminates watching the time tick away when you struggle with fall asleep.

This goes for your cell phone as well. Most phones will light up anytime there is an incoming message or notification. This light can distract you from sleep. If you must have your phone in your bedroom, flip it over so the screen is facing down.

Natural Lights

Using blackout curtains in your room will eliminate natural light. Natural light is necessary in the morning to wake up. Opening up your curtains as soon as you wake can help trigger signals throughout the body. If you do not have blinds or curtains to block out light, try a sleep mask. Sleep masks can make it easier to fall asleep, especially if you share a room.

. . .

SOUNDS

Noise in the bedroom can disrupt your sleep. Sudden noises can lead to frequent awakenings, reducing the length of your sleep. Continuous external noises will also reduce the quality of your sleep.

Sound Machines

Using a white noise machine can help cover up external noises beyond your control. These machines can also deliver a consistent low-frequency sound that will not interrupt your sleep. While external noise does not always contribute to poor sleep, the inconsistency of the sound does. When noise goes from low to high frequencies we are more inclined to wake up. Using a sound machine can help deliver a consistent stream of sound that never fluctuates.

If you are the type of person that likes to fall asleep with music playing, set a timer. Having the music turn off around the time you would typically fall asleep will reduce the inconsistency of the sound that can make it hard to stay asleep.

Guided Sleep

Using a sleep video or sleep recording of a guided meditation can help you fall asleep faster. They can also help improve the quality of your sleep through the night. These videos have a speaker that prompts you into creating certain visuals that will help relax the mind and body. They also provide a peaceful soundtrack of natural sounds that will keep you from thinking too much. There are many videos you can start playing as you lay down for bed. Most display a darker image of a natural setting but others may use a bright sunny beach to help promote a relaxing state. In either case, you want to completely dim your screen, or turn your device away for your bed. While the imagery is nice to look at, you do not want the light from your device keeping you up.

SCENTS

How your bedroom smells will also have an impact on your sleep. While most scents, even if unpleasant, will not cause you to wake up from sleep, a more pleasing smell will make it easier to fall asleep. There are plenty of scents you can use in your bedroom and home to help promote a restful night sleep. Try these aromatherapy scents:

- Lavender
- Chamomile
- Vanilla

- Rose
- Citrus
- Frankincense

You can use one or a combination of scents to help you sleep. Essential oils are great to use on pillows and bedding. Be careful in making sure that they can be used topically so they do not cause skin irritation. You can also use incense or a diffuser which will allow you to have the aroma continuously dispersed throughout your entire room. Additionally, any scent that brings back a pleasing memory or that you just enjoy will improve sleep. Many studies have shown that smelling the scent of your loved one can help you fall asleep faster.

CHAPTER 8 - SLEEP HYGIENE AND HOW TO GET BETTER SLEEP

Sleep hygiene is made up of the right sleep environment and your daily routines. Once you have addressed your sleep environment, it is time to look at the rest of your day. What you do during the day, and not just closer to bedtime, can help you correct poor sleep habits. First, you will learn ways to help track your sleep so you can identify what struggles you are having. Are you not getting enough hours or not getting quality sleep? The rest of the chapter will discuss key lifestyle factors that should be addressed to improve sleep.

TRACKING SLEEP PATTERNS

You may know that you are not getting enough sleep,

but you may not know if it is just a lack of total hours, quality sleep, or a combination that is causing sleep problems. To better find a solution and sleep better you need to start by tracking how you actually sleep.

Duration of Sleep

Track the time you fall asleep and record the time you begin to stir in the morning. This will give you a general idea of how many hours you are asleep during the night. This does not, however, account for all the times you may briefly wake in the evening which impacts your quality of sleep. If you do wake up for longer periods of time you want to keep track of this as well. Fragmented sleep cuts your total hours of sleep, but it can give you a clue as to how much time you are spending in certain sleep cycles. This can also give you a better idea of how much deep sleep versus light sleep you may be getting (National Sleep Foundation, n.d.).

Quality of Sleep

Tracking how often you tend to wake in the evening or when you toss and turn during the night will give you an indication of the quality of sleep you get. Being restless, taking too long to fall asleep, or waking without being able to fall back asleep quickly decreases the quality of your sleep. If you have had a stressful day or notice that you stay awake with racing thoughts, you should keep track of this as well. Since our quality of sleep is directly impacted by our mental well-being, keeping notes daily can help you find the root cause of your poor sleep habits (National Sleep Foundation, n.d.).

Tech Devices That Help

There are plenty of apps and sleep trackers on the market that can help aid in tracking your sleep patterns. One thing to keep in mind about these gadgets is that they often give an estimate on how much time you actually spend asleep. Most devices can pinpoint when you wake up or if you stirred in the night. They can even track environmental changes like room temperature, sounds, and lights, which can contribute to wakefulness. For the most part, however, these trackers cannot measure brain waves which give you a clear indication of your sleep pattern. To measure brain waves while you sleep you would need to undergo a sleep study.

This is not to say that trackers can not provide you with valuable information and help steer you in the right direction for improving sleep. Most trackers will cost up to $100, but they can be used to help track other essential activity during the day as well. Mobile apps, which can be more budget-friendly, can give enough information to help improve your sleep patterns. Some trackers and app to consider include:

- SleepCycle (app)
- FitBit Flex (tracker)
- UP24 Jawbone (tracker)
- Basis (tracker)
- Sleep Time (app)
- Sleep Score (app)
- Motiv Ring (tracker)

Those who suffer from insomnia will benefit more from an alarm clock that keeps track of their sleep cycle. This will allow them to set a time frame for the alarm to go off but will also rely on the alarm clock to set the alarm off when they are not in the middle of REM sleep. This will significantly reduce the tiredness they feel during the day (National Sleep Foundation, 2020). The iPhone also has a similar feature called Bedtime. You set the time you want to go to bed and need to wake up then your phone captures data from when you stop using the device. It also tracks additional data that you can review in their health app under sleep analysis.

.

• • •

Diet

When addressing sleep struggles, diet is usually the last thing one thinks as a contribution to the issue. Sleep and diet, as with many daily activities, go hand in hand. What you eat can affect the quality and duration of your sleep, but your sleep also influences your food choices throughout the day. If you have found it hard to lose weight your sleep might be the reason for this.

A Healthy Sleep Diet

The proper sleep diet is typical of a healthy lifestyle diet. It is rich in whole foods like fresh fruits, vegetables, whole grains, and lean proteins. A healthy sleep diet limits sugar and cuts out processed foods. As a general rule, foods that will cause you to gain weight will interfere with your sleep. This is especially true of what you eat just before you go to bed.

When you do not get the proper sleep in the evening this makes it more likely that you will make poor food choices throughout the day. This causes a negative cycle to occur. When you are sleep deprived, hunger suppressing hormones are not produced when they should be: this causes you to feel hungry even when you are not. When you feel tired, your body will automatically crave sweeter foods to increase energy levels. You are more likely to reach for an unhealthy sweet treat to help combat the cravings. Eating too many high sugar foods causes energy levels to crash midday. You end up feeling more fatigued shortly after the sugar rush which in turn will interrupt your sleep patterns.

When Should Your Last Meal Be?

Eating too late in the day or just before bedtime means your body will still be trying to digest the food you consume while you are asleep. This can increase the chances of suffering from acid reflux, especially if you eat higher fat or spicy foods. Eating a big meal shortly before bedtime causes insulin and cortisol levels to also rise. Even if you happen to fall asleep quickly after a meal, the quality and length of your sleep diminishes.

The general rule is that there should be at least three hours between your last meal and your bedtime. Snacking just before bed can cause sleep disturbances, along with unwanted weight gain. This is because most foods we tend to reach for before bed are processed junk foods that contain high amounts of carbohydrates and sugar (Jones, 2016). You do not, however, want to go to bed hungry. Hunger pains can keep you awake as well. If you find yourself up for longer than three hours after your last big meal, a small piece of fruit or other foods that are quickly digestible are acceptable. You do not want to eat typical junk foods like chips or sweets. Instead, a small piece of fruit like a banana, Greek yogurt, or a small bowl of whole-grain cereal is a much better alternative. Also, avoid drinking caffeine beverages or super sugary drinks as this will increase energy levels rapidly and will make it more difficult to fall asleep.

Foods That Promote a Good Night's Sleep

Fatty Fish/Omega-3's: Fatty fish like salmon provide you with a high dose of omega-3 fatty acids and vitamin D. Both of these are beneficial for overall help, but for sleep they are especially important. They help regulate the body's production of serotonin, the stress hormone that can keep us alert and stressed.

Nuts: Almonds, cashews, and pistachios contain melatonin as well as high amounts of magnesium and zinc. This combination has been shown to help those with insomnia get better sleep.

Lean Protein: Protein that contains tryptophan helps promote sleep. This is an amino acid commonly found in turkey which makes people feel drowsy. When combined with a complex carb like brown or wild rice, you will not only be able to fall asleep faster but stay asleep for longer.

What Should You Drink Before Bed?

Drinking water before bed can combat hunger pains. Most often we feel hungry when in fact we are just thirsty. This, however, can interfere with sleep. If you drink too much water just before bed you may find yourself waking up in the middle of the night to use the restroom. It is better to ensure you are getting enough water throughout the day. Staying hydrated during your daily activities keeps you alert, focused, and can help improve your sleep patterns. When we are dehydrated we feel low on energy causing us to sleep in the middle of the day.

Increasing your water consumption during the day can improve sleep. Cutting back on caffeinated beverages can also help significantly improve sleep, especially if you limit consumption of these beverages to just the morning. Alcohol beverages should be avoided late in the evening as they are shown to increase sleep troubles like snoring and insomnia (National Sleep Foundation, 2020).

In the evening you can choose to drink a warm non-caffeinated beverage like chamomile tea. Tart cherry juice is also a great choice; this gives you something more flavorful to sip on, but it also contains melatonin which will help you fall asleep at bedtime.

•   •   •

EXERCISE

Exercise is the third key component to a healthy life-style. Diet, sleep, and exercise all directly affect the other. Making simple adjusts to your daily routine to include exercise will have a positive impact on sleep. Depending on your physical fitness, age, and overall health, the type of exercise you want to include can vary. For most, just sticking to a consistent exercise plan is all it takes to see significant improvements in sleep. Keep in mind, adding exercise to your routine may increase fatigue during the day. If we are not fueling our body properly with the right foods, we will feel more tired. Learning how to balance diet and exercise to optimize sleep can take time and a bit of trial and error. But, it is one of the best natural ways to correct sleep issues. The good news is that even if you have not figured out the proper diet and exercise routine, even a moderate amount of exercise during your day can help you see positive results quickly.

Exercise promotes a healthy body and mind. It can reduce stress and increase longevity. When it comes to sleep, regular exercise will help you fall asleep faster and increase the length of your sleep. Exercise keeps stress hormones in check by releasing endor-phins, the feel-good chemical.

Best Physical Activity for Better Sleep

Any exercise can improve sleep, but some may do a slightly better job than others. What is important to keep in mind is when you get your exercise in. When we exercise, the feel-good endorphins released can give us a boost in energy. We feel more alert, focused, and awake after exercising. Exercising will also increase the core body temperature. This rise in temperature also sends signals from the brain to the rest of the body that it is time to be awake and ready for the day. Both of these factors can make it difficult to fall asleep if you exercise late in the evening. However, this is not true for everybody, so it is best to experiment with different workout times during the day to see which results in better sleep. Those who suffer from insomnia should get more rigorous exercise during the earlier hours of the day (National Sleep Foundation, 2020).

Aerobic exercise has been shown to increase slow wave brain frequency while you sleep (Bentivoglio & Grassi-Zucconi, 1997). This means you spend more time in deep rejuvenated sleep through the night. Doing a simple stretching routine just before bed will keep the heart rate low and relax the muscles to help promote better sleep.

The important thing about exercising is you do something you enjoy. While aerobics may give you the best results, it will simply not do you any good if you cannot stand doing it and skip your workouts because of it. Strength training, yoga, cycling, running, and dancing can all improve your sleep as well. The goal is to get your heart rate elevated enough to trigger the same response that aerobics does. This is how you improve your sleep.

It is best to try a few different exercises to see which ones you enjoy. You can also switch up what you do during the week to improve your sleep. Tracking what workouts you do and how you sleep through the night can give you a better idea of what works best for you. Also, track when you do these exercises to see what time of the day is best for you to workout to become a better sleeper.

How Often Should You Exercise?

Adding in just 10 to 30 minutes of moderate exercise can help you sleep better that same night. Moderate exercise includes activities like jogging, cycling, and using a treadmill. You want to increase the heart rate slightly, but you should be able to breathe comfortably.

There is no right or wrong answer to how many days you should be exercising. You can incorporate 10 to 20 minutes of aerobic exercises every day to improve sleep or you may find it better to do 20 to 30 minutes at least five days a week. Just as you will want to try out different times for your workout, you will want to switch up how many days you workout during the week.

You can also split up your exercise for optimal results. Try to get in a more vigorous activity in the morning hours to boost energy levels and focus. In the evening, do a light workout like yoga no later than two hours before bed. The littlest bit of exercise can have huge impacts; remember to be consistent and make exercise a daily habit.

STRESS REDUCTION

There is no question that excess stress is going to impair sleep. Stress is one of the leading causes for individuals to suffer from insomnia (National Sleep Foundation, 2020). Troublesome thoughts of things that need to be done, mistakes made, or decisions left undecided all contribute to stress; however, these thoughts are not the only reason we are left wide awake in the late hours. It is not just the big or worrisome thoughts that trigger our stress response. Notification sounds from our phones, watching the news, or listening to a loved one talk about their stressful day can all cause our body to switch to stress mode.

This is why we need to become more mindful and intentional about what we do in the evening hours of our day.

Stress increases cortisol levels, the stress hormone. When these levels remain high, it is more difficult for the body to release relaxation hormones. This leads to a vicious cycle. The more stress you experience, the less sleep you get; the less sleep you get, the more stressed you will feel. If the body does not get the signal to stop producing these hormones, it is impossible for us to fall into deep restorative sleep.

This also has an impact on our overall health. Those who suffer from chronic stress are more at risk of cardiovascular disease, compromised immune system, digestive issues, high blood pressure, and depression. Each of these higher-risk conditions also impairs our sleep (Mayo Clinic, 2019).

Being able to switch on the body's natural relaxation mode is essential for a good night's sleep. But, unwinding before you go to bed isn't the only time you should focus on reducing stress. Performing simple stress-reduction activities can increase the quality and quantity sleep when doing throughout the day or just before bedtime.

. . .

YOGA

There are a variety of yoga practices you can do to help reduce stress. Practicing vinyasa yoga during the day hours keeps stress levels down. This is a type of flow yoga that uses a sequence of poses that we transition to and from based on the breath. Before bed you can utilize similar poses, held for longer, to deliberately put the body into a more relaxed and calm state (Saal, 2019). The poses listed below are ideal because they turn off our fight or flight response, help stretch out and relax tense muscles, and can be done while in bed.

WATERFALL POSE

The waterfall pose—legs up the wall—is great to start off with when you are getting ready for bed. It is also ideal for those who do a lot of sitting or standing during the day as it helps stretch the hamstrings. This pose is considered a slight inversion pose, so the feet are raised above the head. These types of poses further stimulate a relaxed state because they increase blood flow to the brain while slowing down the heart rate.

You can do this pose while lying in bed or on the floor as long as you are positioned close to a wall.

Have a pillow within reach so you can prop yourself up a little more. To perform this pose:

1. Begin in a sitting position facing the wall as close as you can manage.
2. Slowly lower the upper half of the body back as you bring the knees in toward the chest. You can place the feet on the wall.
3. Shift closer to the wall so the sitting bone is an inch or two away, and extend the legs up the wall. If you feel too much pulling in the hamstrings, move a little further away from the wall. The feet should be flat as if you were standing.
4. You can place a pillow just under the lower back for extra support.
5. Hold this pose for 10 breaths. As you inhale, lengthen the stretch in the legs by pressing the feet up further, On the exhale allow your body to relax into the pose; the legs should remain a little firm so they stay extended up against the wall.
6. After 10 breaths, slowly lower the legs and bring the knees back to the chest before returning to your original sitting position.

Twisted Root

You can transition into twisted root from waterfall pose or use this position just before you are ready to sleep. This is a great pose to help with digestion as well. To do this pose:

1. Begin laying on your back with the knees bent and the feet flat on the ground. The feet should be close together.
2. The arms should be at your side with the palms facing down.
3. Keep the shoulders pressed into the ground as you begin to lower the knees to the right side. The upper body should remain in a neutral position.
4. You can bring the left arm up and create a straight line from the right shoulder to the left fingertip to keep the left shoulder grounded.
5. Hold this pose for 10 breaths. On the inhale, allow your hips to fall deeper into the twist as you stretch through the fingertips of the left hand. On the exhale allow yourself to relax into the pose.
6. Once you have held the position for 10 breaths, slowly lift the knees back up and plant the feet back on the ground.

7. Take a deep inhale and slowly exhale before
   lowering the knees to the left side, repeating
   the process as needed.

Child's Pose

Child's pose gives a gentle stretch to the hips and
back, allowing us to fall into a relaxed mind and
body. You can do this pose from your bed: use your
pillows to give you extra support and comfort. To
perform this pose:

1. Begin in a slight tabletop position where the
   hands are planted on the bed or ground just
   under the shoulder blades and knees or on
   the ground in line with the hips.
2. Begin to lower the sit bone toward the heels
   of the feet as you bring the hands to the
   thighs.
3. Open the hips by drawing the knees apart,
   but keep the sit bone resting on the heels of
   the feet.
4. Take a pillow, and rest it on the thighs. Begin
   to fold forward so the chest rests on the
   pillow. Stretch the arms out in front of you
   with the palms facing down. You can turn the

head to one side or let the forehead rest
gently on the ground.

5. Hold this position for 10 breaths. As you
    inhale, allow the sitting bone to sink deeper
    toward the heels as the arms extend further
    out above the head. On the exhale, allow the
    body to relax into the pose.

6. After 10 breaths, slowly lift the chest up off
    the floor back into your original sitting
    position.

Meditation

Meditation has been proven to lower stress levels,
but any gentle breathing exercises will help you
relax. Many have misconceptions about what meditation entails. You do not need a super quiet zen space
—though it might not hurt to try—you do not need
to dedicate 30 or more minutes a day, and you
certainly do not need to do it perfectly every time.
There is not a one-size-fits-all for mediation; luckily,
there are many different techniques that you can try.
Meditation is something you can easily do from
anywhere: while at your desk at work, in the kitchen
of your home, while walking in the park, or sitting
quietly in your bedroom before bed.

· · ·

DEEP BREATHING

Deep breathing is a meditation technique that can be done from anywhere and anytime. This type of meditation requires you to focus on your breathing—taking a deep inhale, filling the abdomen, and slowly exhaling. At any time during your day, you can dim the lights, and sit for a few deep breaths. Focus intently on how the air fills you as you inhale for a count of three to five, pausing for a second, then slowly exhaling for another count of three to five. This can also be done while lying in bed. Place your hands on your abdomen, and focus on how your hands rise and lower with your breath.

MINDFULNESS

Mindfulness meditation is a great technique that teaches you to acknowledge any troublesome thoughts but not dwell on them. It is a way for you to slow down your thought process so you focus on one thing at a time and then let it go. Letting go is an important aspect of mindfulness meditation. It is a way to keep yourself aligned with the present moment instead of getting caught up with anxiety of the past or worries of the future (Bertone, 2020).

Like all other meditations, mindfulness can be practiced at any time. You can practice while you are eating: shift your focus to how the food you are eating tastes, smells, and satisfies you. You can bring more awareness in the middle of your day by shifting your focus to your senses as you walk to your car or wait to pick the kids up from school. Even taking a moment to just pause, breathe, and then react to external stimulants gives you enough time to slow down, like pausing before you answer your phone when it rings or sounds with a new notification.

Before bed, you can tame your stressful thoughts with mindful meditation. As you lay in bed, bring your attention first to breathe. Do not try to control your breath—instead allow yourself to fall into a naturally inhale/exhale pattern. Then choose a phrase to repeat it yourself—"I am calm," "I am relaxed," or "I welcome sleep" are all good options. Begin to repeat this phrase as you allow the body to relax more and more. Your thoughts will try to pull your attention—acknowledge your thoughts. Simply stating or "thinking" out loud will remind you to shift your focus back to the present moment and on your calming phrases (Bertone, 2020).

Journaling

Getting concerns out of your head can help you switch your brain to off mode. Jot down the things that are taking up energy and pulling at your attention away from sleep. Then set the list aside and address these concerns in the morning. Journaling helps put your thoughts to bed, so to speak. It also gives us the opportunity to slow down. We can write down our out of control thoughts and a more organized manner. Doing this provides us with the chance to see what we are thinking from a new perspective, one that does not have to be stressful or cause anxiety.

Day Journal

You simply cannot do much late at night with the thoughts that are running through your mind. Practicing writing down any of your issues in a journal during the day will help you give it better attention during the day hours than in the evening hours where nothing can be done with them except rob you of your sleep.

Gratitude Journal

Gratitude has a way of helping us see the best we already have. It reminds us that even though we may have worries, we have so much more to be thankful for. This gets us in the habit of developing a more positive mindset which benefits us in more ways than just helping with sleep.

Before bed, list three things that made you smile that day. These can be any small or big detail. Did someone pay for your coffee in the morning? Was the sun shining most of the day? Did you get that promotion? Maybe you are just thankful that you woke up in good health. Any three things, list them each night.

Pause and look around you, find one thing that you value most in the moment.

1. List one relationship you are grateful for. Why?
2. List three things you like about yourself that day.
3. What was one thing you learned that week, month, or year that has helped you grow?

BEDTIME JOURNAL PROMPTS TO GET YOU STARTED

1. In the evening you can write about one positive experience from the day. Go into detail about what happened and how it made you feel.

2. Write out your to-do list before bed. This gets all the anxious feeling of what you need to do out. When you have your list you will not fear forgetting or keep yourself in an overwhelming position.
3. What is your fondest memory?
4. What is one negative experience you are holding onto? What do you need to do to let this go?
5. What is one thing you are looking forward to tomorrow?
6. What are five things you can do to make yourself feel better when you are upset, disappointed, stressed, or sad?
7. Describe one place you would love to visit. How can you make that trip happen? How would it make you feel?
8. What is the best advice you ever received?
9. What is one small thing you can begin to do in the morning that will help you achieve a big goal or change an unpleasant situation?
10. What do I want to dream about tonight?

Self-Care

Sleep should be a part of your self-care routine; many of the other items discussed in this chapter also contribute to self-care.

It is hard to do things for yourself, whether that is getting enough zzz's or taking 30 minutes to enjoy a hobby. We get caught up in feeling that if we are not doing something directly for others then we are being selfish. Self-care is a selfless act. You cannot give enough energy, focus, and affection to others if you are not giving yourself the same thoughts and considerations.

Self-care can take on many forms. It can be a trip to a spa or creating a spa day in your own home with a steamy bubble bath and scented candles. It can also be a relaxing weekend by yourself in the mountains or a quiet afternoon in the park. It can be splurging on a new pair of shoes or blocking out an hour to write or paint. Whatever you do, take the time to do what makes you feel good.

This makes you feel more fulfilled; the activities you decide to do will eliminate stress. This means you not only will get better sleep, but you are more motivated and able to do more for others.

Napping

Sometimes naps are a necessity. When you are sick, your body needs more rest. When you are stressed, feeling anxious, or have unexpected sleep disturbances, naps can help keep your circadian rhythm in sync. Naps can also remove some of your sleep debt.

Napping for long hours or later in the day will interfere with your evening sleep cycle though. If you need to nap, take one early in the day. Naps should be short: they are just a pause to give the rest of your body time to recoup. A 20 to 30 minute power nap should be sufficient enough to refuel your energy levels. Longer naps that are 60 to 90 minutes long can also be rejuvenating, but only if they occur early in the afternoon hours. Taking a longer nap like this later in the day will make it harder to fall asleep in the evening (Suni, 2020).

AFFECTION

As humans we naturally crave affection. It helps us feel protected, cared for, and happy, but affection can also have a positive impact on your sleep. When we hug or kiss our body's release oxytocin, they feel a good chemical that makes us feel calm and in control. Receiving affection also makes us feel supported. This results in our stress levels being reduced twice: one from the release of oxytocin and second from feeling supported (Penn Medicine, 2018).

To maintain the positive benefits of affection we

should strive to get in at least eight hugs a day. This can be quite challenging for most people as we are always on the go. However, getting in a few hugs is better than none at all. Cuddling with your partner in the evening can also cause the same chemical reactions which can make it easier to fall asleep.

Keep in mind, this correlates to how responsive your partner is to your needs outside of the bedroom. Cuddling up to someone when we do not have a strong connection to them may not give us the same sleep benefits we desire. To fall into the deep restorative sleep that helps us feel refreshed and full of energy the next day, we need to feel a sense of safety and security when we sleep next to someone.

CHAPTER 9 - FALL ASLEEP FASTER

Even those who have regular sleep patterns can struggle to get to sleep sometimes. Whether it is due to stress, extra to-do's to complete before bed, or life curveballs that dip into your sleep time, it is important to be able to adapt and get the sleep you need. To do this, you need to have an arsenal of tips and tricks that will help you fall asleep faster no matter what has occurred throughout your day. In this chapter, you will learn various techniques that will help you get to sleep and stay asleep for longer. Even if you have struggled with insomnia or sleep disturbance, you are sure to find a go-to method to improve your quality and quantity of sleep.

. . .

Fall Asleep in 30 Minutes or Less

Falling asleep in less than 30 minutes is a sign of good sleep hygiene. For most, we toss and turn for much longer than that when we finally get into bed. Establishing the right routine in the evening can help you fall asleep faster. Performing the right activities at bedtime will also make falling asleep easier.

Evening Routine

Create an evening routine that gets you in the mood to sleep—dim the lights, lower the temperature, and get comfortable. Your evening routine is vital for getting your mind and body in the mood for sleep. We have already discussed thoroughly how to set up your environment as well as some before bed activities to ensure better sleep; now it is time to create an actual routine and commit to it. When creating your routine remember:

1. Eat your last big meal three hours before bedtime.
2. Turn off electronics at least an hour before hitting your bed.
3. Do one thing that relaxes the body—take a warm bath or do some yoga.
4. Do something that relaxes the mind— meditation or reading.

5. Do something to get your thoughts ready for bed—journaling or writing a to-do list

6. Spend quality time with your partner or children.

7. Call a relative or close friend.

You can add as many activities to your evening routine as you wish.

Prep Your Environment

When it starts getting closer to the time you want to sleep, begin prepping your environment. Be sure electronics are off, your alarm is set and turned away from you, and you have everything you need ready for the next day. Going through the motion of preparing your bed for sleep you can begin to train your brain to associate these actions with sleep. When done consistently, you will begin to feel more tired when you go through the motions of prepping your environment: this will result in you falling asleep faster.

Begin by dimming the lights and shutting the curtains 30 minutes before you plan to fall asleep. Lower the temperature in your room so your body gets in sleep mode. If you need a sound machine turn it on, but keep the volume low and just barely audible. Then take up to 10 minutes to journal, followed by around 10 minutes of reading. Choose something that only slightly intrigues you to read; for better sleep, the more boring it is to read, the sleepier it will make you. If you are not already laying in bed, lay down and do breathing exercises. Try the 4-7-8 method (Legg, 2019):

1. Press your tongue to the back of your top teeth and inhale for a count of four through the nose.
2. Hold your breath for a count of seven, keep the tongue pressed on the back teeth.
3. Exhale for a count of eight through the mouth.
4. Repeat until you fall asleep.

Brian Dump

Doing an evening brain dump can be considered a form of journaling but with less structure. While journaling can be done in your bed to shift to a positive mindset, a brain dump should be done a little earlier to your bedtime. The purpose is to get all the thoughts and ideas out of your head so you are not trying to plan or further examine them when you lay down. When doing a brain dump you want to get everything out of your head. Not surprisingly, when you go to sit down and write all the things down, your brain will suddenly hit a wall. All of a sudden you may not have anything to write, and you celebrate thinking you will be able to go to sleep soundly without the racing thoughts: that is until you lie down and they appear. To help combat this, work through specific categories. You can dedicate a page in a notebook to each, or just keep a short list handy to refer to when you get stuck. Some categories to consider:

- Work-related thoughts and tasks
- Family
- Healthy
- Finances
- Upcoming deadline or appointments you need to make
- Grocery/shopping lists
- Things that need to be done in the home
- Things that need to be fixed or replaced
- Personal goals
- Meal planning
- Volunteering or community work
- People you should call
- Questions you keep asking yourself
- Additional ideas

Once you have your list, if you find that there are some things you want to expand on, then write down a few words or short phrases. This list is not a get it out and forget it list, otherwise, the same thoughts will keep creeping in night after night. Instead, you want to be sure to look over this list in the morning. Then pick one or two things to cross off the list that day. You will not be able to cross everything off your list, and many of the items will just be random thoughts—not necessarily things to do. This creates a system to help alleviate anxiety. Just doing the brain dump will lead to feeling like you are wasting time, overwhelmed, or that you need to get started on the list the night you make it: this is not what we want to occur. When you utilize the list and look it over, you are giving it more purpose, your brain begins to trust the process, and you get more done.

Try to do your brain dump outside of the bedroom. When you are done, close your notebook and then go on with your regular evening routine. This will already have begun the process of getting your mind ready to sleep. A brain dump can be the trigger activity you do that starts your bedtime routine which trains the brain to perform the task and shut off.

． ． ．

FALL ASLEEP IN 60 SECONDS OR LESS

If you suffer from onset insomnia you want to have additional tricks handy to help you fall asleep as quickly as possible. While falling asleep too quickly on your own can be a result of sleep deprivation, if you toss and turn or have racing thoughts when you lay down, you need to have a plan in place to help you fall asleep fast. The following techniques combine deep breathing and shifting the focus of your thoughts. This leads to being able to relax the body and mind in no time, so you can fall asleep without tossing and turning.

Muscle Relaxation

Progressive muscle relaxation combines deep breathing, targeted muscle tightening and relaxation, and mindfulness in one exercise. Though the whole process can take longer than 60 seconds, most find they fall asleep shortly after beginning. Once you are laying down comfortably in bed close the eyes then go through the following steps:

1. Take a few deep breaths.
2. Starting at the toes—with the dominant side of the body—begin to tense the muscle. Start with the toes, then the feet; after this, move up the legs and thighs. Keeping the dominant

side tense, repeat the process on your non-dominant leg.

3. Once the muscles in both legs are tense, continue with the hips, lower back, then the shoulder.
4. Starting with the dominant arm, begin to tense the muscle of the upper arm, then the forearm, wrist, and fingers. Once all the muscles are tense on the dominant side, move to the non-dominant side.
5. Keeping the lower body tense begins to tense the muscle of the neck and face.
6. After reaching the top of your head, keep the whole body tense for three breaths.
7. Begin to slowly untense the muscle in reverse until you reach the toes, once again on your dominant side.

You may not get through the whole process which is what we want. As you go through the tense of your muscles, it can help to keep your thoughts focused on the process. When you tense a muscle group take note of any aches or pains you may feel, but do not dwell on them. Simply tell yourself that these muscles can rest and repair now. Some also find it helpful to say a few words of gratitude to specific areas. If you have a demanding job that requires you to be on your feet most of the day, as you tense the muscle of your feet and legs, you can thank them for carrying you through the day.

Variations

Some find it easier to go through a section of the body instead of doing a full-body relaxation. You can do this by choosing an area that feels especially tense, like the legs, shoulders, or neck. Tense the muscle and keep them tense for 10 breaths then gently relax the muscles before moving onto the next section.

Visualizations

Using visualization can help you relax and fall asleep fast. We already discussed how using guided meditation can soothe you into a peaceful state; visualization can be performed without guidance. To use visualization, begin to think of a quiet and calm place. This can vary, though—most use a sandy beach as their ending destination while others like to take a more realistic approach using a familiar setting. For this example we will use the sandy beach setting. The goal is to bring to mind as much detail as you can. This example is laid out to give you a general idea of what you should picture as well as asking key questions to help you draw out more details of your own visualization.

First, picture yourself at the top of a sand dune that

leads down to a white sandy beach. What are you wearing? How does the sun feel on your skin? Bring into focus the crashing waves. Just up from the shore-line, you spot a hammock nestled between two tall palm trees. No one else is around. You hear the gentle rolling of water and rustle of sand. What else do you hear? You begin to slowly descend down the sand dune. How does the breeze feel on your face? How does the sand feel under your feet? You reach the bottom of the sand dune and look around. You look up to see a clear blue sky. Do you see any clouds? If so, do any of them form a specific shape or object? You begin to walk towards the hammock. When you reach the hammock, you lay down in it. How does it feel to be swinging freely, completely relaxed? Close your eyes. Do you still hear the waves crashing on the beach? Are their birds chirping in the distance?

Stressful Day

When you are experiencing higher levels of stress there are techniques you can utilize before bed to help ward off troublesome thoughts. We have discussed how important it is to incorporate stress reduction practices into your day, but sometimes you need a little extra help in the evening. To help combat high levels of stress and help you fall asleep faster, the following exercises can be effective.

Diaphragmatic Breathing

Diaphragmatic breathing is a deep breathing technique used to control breathing and slow the heart rate. This exercise utilizes counting backward to keep your thoughts better focused and bring a more calm and relaxed state to the mind and body.

Begin laying down in your bed. Prop up the knees slightly by placing a pillow under them. Place a hand on your chest and the other on your stomach. Inhale and exhale slowly through your nose. Notice how your hands rise and fall with your breath. Repeat this three times, then inhale and exhale through the mouth. Again, watch as the hands rise and fall with your breath. Continue to breathe in and out until you notice the hand on your chest does not rise. Now begin to count backward from 10. When you hit zero, inhale and exhale through the nose again and repeat the process. Take note if the hand on your chest raises after you have counted back from 10. Repeat a total of three times.

Body Scan

A body scan is a type of mindfulness meditation practice that helps you locate tension in the body and release it. Using this technique near bedtime can lead to a better night's sleep as you will feel like you are carrying around less stress for the day. For stress and anxiety especially, you can release tension you did not even realize you were carrying around. This keeps you better in tune with physical signs your body gives you that lets you know you are feeling overly stressed.

A full-body scan can take up to 10 minutes to thoroughly perform. You can sit in a comfortable chair or lay in bed; however, this practice should not be used to fall asleep, so a comfortable chair is better suited.

1. Begin in a sitting position.
2. Slowly close your eyes.
3. Bring your focus on how your body feels. How does your body feel sitting in the chair or lying in bed? Where are your hands positioned? How do they feel where they are? Are your legs crossed or stretched out in front of you? How do they feel in this position? As you quickly check in with how your overall body feels, keep your breath steady—taking a deep inhale and slow exhale.
4. Next, start at the feet. How do they feel? Are there any areas that tingle, throb, or feel

pain? If you do not have any sensation coming from the feet, that is fine as well. Take note of the sensation then move on to the legs. Again, pay attention to any pains, twitches, or tension. Work your way to the legs, stopping for just a few seconds to take notice of any sensations you may be feeling. Continue this process of acknowledging the sensations your body is giving off as you slowly work all the way to the crown of your head.

5. If you notice your thoughts have distracted you from the sensation of your body, this is completely expected. When you do notice this happening just bring your attention back to a particular body part and continue.

6. Once you have reached the crown of your head, take a minute or more to bring your awareness back to how your whole body feels. Take a few more deep breaths before you slowly open your eyes.

Self-Hypnosis

Hypnosis brings us to a deeply relaxed state. It is a practice that can take time to master, but even when just starting out, the results can lead to a longer and more restful sleep. It can be beneficial to use an app or guided hypnosis recording to help you enter into a trance-like state that helps you fall asleep faster.

There are many variations for how to perform a sleep self-hypnosis. Some utilize water such as rain or a shower falling that progressively rises around you until your body is completely submerged in the water. Others use metaphors like a fish diving deep into the ocean water. You may want to try a few different types of self-hypnosis to see which allows you to get into a deeply relaxed state. For this example, we will use a deep diving setting as it better symbolizes diving deeper into sleep. It is best to perform a self-hypnosis after you have done a body relaxation technique such as the progressive muscle relaxation described earlier in this chapter. When the body is more relaxed it can be easier to get the mind into a deeper state of sleep through self-hypnosis. While the steps may appear to be done rather quickly it is important to take each step slowly. Once you read over them you will be able to perform the hypnosis at your own pace, and each step should not be rushed.

1. Begin laying in your bed. Lay in your typical sleeping position; if you toss and turn choose the most comfortable position at the time.

Keep in mind you will not want to move at all through the entire hypnosis.

2. Visualize yourself standing in shallow water at a beach. The water is just covering your feet. Pause and let your feet relax as the water covers them.

3. You take a step forward and the water rises to the ankles. Pause and let the ankles relax as the water rises above them.

4. When you take another step the water is halfway up the shins. With another step the water raises around the knees, then the thighs, until it is up to your waist. Your legs are feeling light as the water continues to rise with each step taken. Continue to slowly take a step forward and take notice of the water rising around you.

5. Once the water is about neck high, your body should feel completely relaxed, allow yourself to lay back and float along the water. Feel the water carrying you out to sea, completely relaxed.

6. Now allow yourself to dive under the water. As you dive deeper, see the water becoming darker. Imagine yourself as a little fish diving deeper and deeper into the ocean. Allow the coolness of the water to relax your arms and

legs, so it is completely effortless for you to swim further down.

7. As you continue to dive deeper, allow your mind to slow down and relax. The further you dive in with your visualization, the further you dive into sleep.

If you have gone through all the steps and still find yourself awake, or if you noticed your thoughts have carried you away from the hypnosis, that is fine. Slowly count to five and start over. You will repeat the process a second time and fall asleep quickly.

SLEEP STIMULANTS AND MEDICATIONS

Many people rely on sleeping pills or medication to help them fall asleep. While these aids may help you feel groggy and help you drift to sleep they should not be used as a substitute for getting your body on its own natural sleep cycle. These aids can temporarily help you sleep, but they act as sedatives. When one is sedated the brain is unable to properly switch its frequencies as you sleep. This also makes it more difficult to transition from a stable sleep to a more alert state of wakefulness.

Most over-the-counter sleep aids contain diphenhydramine or doxylamine succinate, two antihistamines commonly used to treat allergies. These ingredients are found in drugs like Benadryl. While they will make you feel drowsy, using an over-the-counter sleep aid should be used infrequently: no more than two weeks at a time. Individuals who have other medical conditions should speak to their doctor before trying over-the-counter medications like these (Mayo Clinic Staff, 2019). Those with a family history of dementia should avoid antihistamines as they increase the risk further of developing dementia. Additionally, those with heart disease, high blood pressure, kidney issues, or liver issues would also steer clear of using sleep aids (Mayo Clinic Staff, 2019).

WAKING UP EARLIER

Many people opt to sleep in when they struggle with sleep. While you want to get enough sleep each night, sleeping in too late will make it difficult to fall asleep in the evening. Instead of sleeping in, get to bed earlier. As we mentioned earlier, pushing up your bedtime by 15 minutes can make this easier to adjust to. By getting to bed earlier you will be able to wake up at a reasonable time that will not have an impact on getting to sleep later. Waking up earlier can make it easier to fall asleep at night since you are starting your day earlier; you will want to sleep earlier as well.

Adjusting your waking time can help regulate your natural rhythm; this also helps with the body's natural melatonin release (National Sleep Foundation, n.d.). As with most other methods, you want to ease into an earlier bedtime. Begin by setting your alarm for just 10 or 15 minutes earlier. Keep this new wake up time for a few days. If you still are struggling to get to bed at a reasonable hour, bump up your wake time another 15 minutes. Continue to do this until you have adjusted your wake and sleep time that allows you to get the proper hours of sleep with the least amount of effort.

CHAPTER 10 - SLEEP THERAPY

If getting enough sleep continues to be a struggle, it may be time for additional outside help. Most people think that they need to struggle with sleep on their own. They obtain a mindset that their poor sleep is just something they need to deal with, and there is little to be done. This is especially true of individuals who have suffered for months or years of sleep issues. There are alternative methods and treatments available for sleep problems. Therapy has been an effective form of treatment for individuals with insomnia. In this final chapter, we will cover additional options for you to get better sleep.

. . .

Seeing a Sleep Specialist

If you find that no matter what steps you take to get more restorative sleep you are still feeling exhausted throughout the day, you will want to speak to your doctor. While feeling tired during the day every once in a while is normal, when you constantly feel fatigued, this can be the result of a more serious sleep disorder.

If all else has failed, it is time to seek out additional help to figure out the reason you are not sleeping. A sleep specialist can help you identify and find a solution to help you get the quality sleep you need. There are a few different types of sleep specialists. Some doctors go through special training in sleep medicine to receive additional certification in sleep treatments. Sleep psychologists are individuals who address mental and behavioral issues that cause sleep disturbances. Otolaryngologists—ear, nose, and throat doctors—are specialists that address issues with the nose, mouth, ears, or throat that are making it difficult to sleep properly. There are many other sleep specialists that specialize in specific areas from nervous disorders to pediatrics.

You should consider seeing a sleep specialist if you:

- Snore

- Have difficulty breathing when you sleep
- Trouble falling asleep
- Wake up frequently through the night
- Feel exhausted through the day no matter how much sleep you got the night before
- Your exhaustion is interfering with your daily activities

When you see a sleep specialist you will need to go through some sleep studies so they see your sleep pattern. This will give them a better idea of when your sleep is being disrupted and may also find what is causing the disruptions. After the test, they may give you a diagnosis. From there, you can discuss further testing that needs to be done, treatment options, and additional lifestyle changes you should make to improve your conditions.

Whether you have been trying to improve your sleep on your own or have struggled with sleep for a prolonged period of time, it is always reassuring to get a professional opinion. Seeing a sleep specialist can better help you take the necessary steps to get you to sleep.

Cognitive Behavioral Therapy

Those who suffer from insomnia can benefit greatly

from Cognitive Behavioral Therapy (CBT). Because insomnia is directly associated with high levels of stress and/or anxiety, this type of treatment addresses the root problem of your stress and anxiety which results in sleep improvements. It also addresses the mindset you have about sleep and your inability to fall asleep or stay asleep, so you can welcome sleep every night in a more positive way (Suni, 2020).

CBT does not just address the symptoms—not falling asleep quickly or waking frequently. It also does not provide generic quick fixes. It treats the core problems of sleep so that you can develop a healthy sleep pattern for the long term. The combination of cognitive and behavioral therapy tackles the main components that cause insomnia and other sleep disorders.

You will learn how to recognize and change the negative thoughts or beliefs you have around sleep. Then, you learn how to avoid behaviors that tend to keep you tossing and turning all night. These behaviors are replaced with more positive actions that result in deeper, more relaxed sleep.

How Can It Help Improve Sleep?

CBT helps you identify sleep-related behaviors that contribute to your insomnia. These include:

- Correcting habits that were once used to improve sleep but over time have become ineffective
- Addressing worrisome thoughts that increase anxiety around sleep
- Conditioned arousal or strengthen the connection that the bedroom is for sleep and not for alertness

Working with a trained therapist can help guide you to taking action in overcoming the obstacles that impair your sleep. The changes that are made have the most significant impact on sleep, which result in being able to see improvement after only a few sessions. For most patients, the notice improves after just two or four sessions, but others may need a little longer to see consistent results.

You will also learn effective relaxation techniques that are specifically catered to help what you are struggling with the most. Your therapist will also guide you to find the appropriate lifestyle changes you should implement to better your sleep. Additionally, CBT can help address the emotional trigger that causes you to lose sleep like anxiety, depression, and stress (Suni, 2020).

. . .

HOLISTIC/NATURAL SLEEP AIDS

Aside from the suggestions and tips discussed in Chapters 7 and 8, there are a few other ways you can naturally improve your sleep. These range from various supplements to various alternative medicine treatments. In this chapter, you will find a few other sleep aids you might want to try that are all natural and have helped others get a better night's sleep.

Supplements to Try

Melatonin: Melatonin is the most widely known natural sleep aid that most people try first. Since this is a naturally produced chemical in the body that is necessary to promote long quality sleep, it is also the most popular. There are other supplements that you can try either on their own or while also taking melatonin to improve your sleep.

Magnesium: Magnesium is a vital mineral the body needs to perform several processes in the body, one of which is melatonin production. This mineral is also responsible for increasing levels of gamma aminobutyric acid (GABA) in the brain. GABA promotes a calming effect in the brain. It is also shown to relax the muscles in the body leading to more quality longer sleep.

Magnesium is found naturally in a variety of foods such as whole grains, low-fat dairy, green vegetables, dry beans, and nuts. Incorporating more of these foods into your diet can remove the need for a supplement.

Valerian Root: This root is native to Europe and Asia. It has been used to help treat anxiety and depression, but has also helped improve quality of sleep in many. It, however, is not meant to be taken for the long-term. Those wishing to try this supplement should do so sparingly.

Vitamin B: Taking a vitamin B supplement along with magnesium and melatonin has been shown to help those with insomnia. Vitamin B can further help regulate our sleep/wake cycle and help us fall into deeper restorative sleep.

Vitamin D: Most people suffer from a vitamin D deficiency, so it is no surprise that most people also struggle with getting good quality sleep. Vitamin D has been shown to help regulate mood, improve bone health, and support the immune system, especially with inflammation control. Vitamin D is also crucial to regulating our sleep/wake circadian rhythm. Natural sunlight is the best source for our body to get vitamin D which is also how our body becomes alert and shifts from sleep mode to alert mode. Increasing vitamin D levels can help improve the quality and length of sleep.

Like melatonin, most of these supplements do come with minor side effects such as headaches, nausea, dizziness that subsides through the day, and diarrhea (Petre, 2020).

Alternative Medicines

Many of the lifestyle changes are natural alternatives that can be used to improve sleep, such as those mentioned in Chapter 8. Yoga and meditation are two of the best alternative medicines to improve sleep, but there are a few others you might be interested in. Unlike yoga and meditation, which can be done daily, this option should be done on an as-needed basis.

ACUPUNCTURE

Acupuncture has been used in the Eastern world to help treat sleep issues for centuries. This type of treatment targets specific points in the body to stimulate various nerves and muscles while also improving blood flow. This stimulation helps relieve pain, stress, anxiety, and other issues that contribute to sleep disturbances. It also helps balance and restore our natural energy levels which makes us feel more calm, clear-headed, and in control. The treatment does use tiny needles but is painless. Just undergoing one session can help you sleep better that same night, though multiple sessions will lead to better results.

MASSAGE

Treating yourself to a massage at least once a month can help you see sleep improvements. Massage helps you gain mental clarity while also relaxing the muscles in the body. It is the perfect way to balance calming the mind and body. What is also beneficial is that this type of alternative treatment can help break up tense and tight muscles that contribute to stress, pain, and poor quality of sleep. You will find that when you regularly schedule in different types of massages you will see an increase in the quality and quantity of sleep you enjoy.

When you do not have the time or extra funds to go to a massage specialist, or if you want to incorporate massage more regularly into your day, you can invest in a foam roller. Foam rollers are commonly used to help athletes relieve muscle strain and pain. They can also be an effective and budget-friendly way to help you get better sleep.

CONCLUSION

Poor sleep is a common struggle that can have a serious impact on every area of your life. You know what it is like to drag your feet and feel out of control because you are too tired to remain alert and present. While this has been your normal up until now, it does not have to be any longer.

You no longer have to lay awake wishing yourself to sleep. The nights of constantly tossing and turning can be part of your past. The sleep aids and other ineffective substances you have used to fall asleep faster will no longer be necessary. Now you have all the information and tools to help set your life up for better sleep.

Improving your sleep begins by gaining the understanding of your own internal clock. You now know how much sleep you need each night to feel refreshed and energized for the next day. Making it a priority to get the adequate hours of sleep will take some changes, but remember: you cannot force yourself to function properly on less sleep than what your body needs. We can, however, train ourselves to have better sleep.

You can recover from your sleep debt and get yourself on a proper schedule. This book has shown you how to set up your environment so that your mind and body feel more relaxed in bed. Remember, treat your bedroom as a sleep sanctuary. The bedroom should be used primarily for sleep. Other activities like watching movies and working should be kept out of the bedroom. It is important to shift how you look at your bedroom in this way. What you do more often in your bedroom is what your brain will associate that room with. Get into the habit of looking at your bedroom as a place for peaceful sleep, and you will find it easier to fall asleep.

You have also realized that the sleep habits you have established over the months and years are no longer serving you. It takes commitment to get into a new routine with your sleep, but the time spent on adjusting your sleep routine is well spent and an investment in your health and happiness for the future.

I hope that the information in this book provides you with the solutions to tackle your biggest sleep worries. I also hope you now have the confidence and understanding that quality sleep is possible. If you take the time to enjoy the time you spend sleeping and look at it as a way to improve the other areas of your life, you will no longer sacrifice sleep. Instead, you will establish better routines in your day to ensure your sleep is not interrupted in the evening. When you learn to look at sleep as a tool to increase your productivity and add value to your life, you will treat it as an essential instead of a second-rate prize for getting through your day. Instead of treating sleep as an option, you will look at it as a need: a need that you will not let other activities intrude on or thoughts that waste your time.

Now that you know the steps to take to get better sleep, it is time to experience it for yourself. I hope you have many restful nights!

REFERENCES

Bentivoglio, M., & Grassi-Zucconi, G. (1997). *The pioneering experimental studies on sleep deprivation.* Sleep, 20(7), 570–576. https://pubmed.ncbi.nlm.nih.gov/9322273/

Bhaskar, S., Hemavathy, D., & Prasad, S. (2016). Prevalence of chronic insomnia in adult patients and its correlation with medical comorbidities. *Journal of Family Medicine and Primary Care,* 5(4), 780–784.

www.ncbi.nlm.nih.gov/pmc/articles/PMC5353813/

Cafasso, J. (2018, September 18). Sleeping with Eyes Open: Treatment and Causes. Retrieved January 12, 2021, from https://www.healthline.com/health/sleeping-with-eyes-open

Committee on Sleep Medicine and Research. (n.d.).

Sleep Disorders and Sleep Deprivation: An Unmet Public Health Problem. In www.nap.edu. https://www.nap.edu/read/11617/chapter/1#

de Bellefonds, C. (2020, February 19). What Is Sleep Regression? Retrieved January 12, 2021, from https://www.whattoexpect.com/first-year/sleep/sleep-regression/

Gniazdowski, L. (2019, July 16). *How to choose a pillow.* Best Health Magazine Canada. https://www.besthealthmag.ca/best-you/home-and-family/how-to-choose-a-pillow/.

Green, E. (2020, June 22). *10 Sleep Deprivation Experiments: Records, Science & Torture.* No Sleepless Nights. https://www.nosleeplessnights.com/sleep-deprivation-experiments

Healthy Sleep. (n.d.). *Sleep, Learning, and Memory Healthy Sleep.* Harvard.Edu. http://healthysleep.med.harvard.edu/healthy/matters/benefits-of-sleep/learning-memory

Jones, T. (2016, October 28). *Is Eating Before Bed Good for You, or Bad?* Healthline. https://www.healthline.com/nutrition/eating-before-bed.

Leavitt, J. (2019, October 10). How Much Deep Sleep Do You Need? Retrieved January 12, 2021, from https://www.healthline.com/health/how-much-deep-sleep-do-you-need

Legg, T. J. (2019, February 12). *4-7-8 breathing: How it works, benefits, and uses*. Medical News Today. https://www.medicalnewstoday.com/articles/324417.

LeWine, H. (2014). *Too little sleep, and too much, affect memory*. Harvard Health Blog. https://www.health.harvard.edu/blog/little-sleep-much-affect-memory-20140502713

Mayo Clinic Staff. (2019, October 16). *Your guide to over-the-counter sleep aids*. Mayo Clinic. https://www.mayoclinic.org/healthy-life-style/adult-health/in-depth/sleep-aids/art-20047860.

Mayo Clinic. (2019, March 19). *Chronic stress puts your health at risk*. Mayo Clinic. https://www.mayoclinic.org/healthy-lifestyle/stress-management/in-depth/stress/art-20046037.

Mayo Clinic. (2020, January 21). Restless legs syndrome. Retrieved January 12, 2021, from https://www.mayoclinic.org/diseases-conditions/restless-legs-syndrome/symptoms-causes/syc-20377168

Mayo Clinic. (2020, July 28). *Sleep apnea*. Mayo Clinic. https://www.mayoclinic.org/diseases-conditions/sleep-apnea/diagnosis-treatment/drc-20377636.

Mayo Clinic. (2020, November 6). *Narcolepsy*. Mayo Clinic. https://www.mayoclinic.org/diseases-conditions/narcolepsy/symptoms-causes/syc-20375497.

National Sleep Foundation. (2015, February 2). *National Sleep Foundation Recommends New Sleep Times.* National Sleep Foundation. Sleepfoundation.org. https://www.sleepfoundation.org/press-release/national-sleep-foundation-recommends-new-sleep-time

National Sleep Foundation. (2020, December 11). What Causes Insomnia? Retrieved January 12, 2021, from https://www.sleepfoundation.org/insomnia/what-causes-insomnia

National Sleep Foundation. (2020, December 12). Infographic: Electronics and Sleep in the Modern Family. Retrieved January 12, 2021, from https://www.sleepfoundation.org/how-sleep-works/infographic-electronics-and-sleep-modern-family

National Sleep Foundation. (2020, October 27). How Are Night Terrors Different from Nightmares. Retrieved January 12, 2021, from https://www.sleep-.org/what-is-a-night-terror/

National Sleep Foundation. (2021, January 08). Anxiety and Sleep. Retrieved January 12, 2021, from https://www.sleepfoundation.org/mental-health/anxiety-and-sleep

National Sleep Foundation. (2021, January 09). Excessive Sleepiness. Retrieved January 12, 2021, from https://www.sleepfoundation.org/excessive-sleepiness

National Sleep Foundation. (n.d.). *How to Get Rid of All of Your Sleep Debt and Feel Well Rested Again.* Sleep.org. https://www.sleep.org/say-goodbye-sleep-debt

National Sleep Foundation. (n.d.). *Relaxation Exercises for Falling Asleep.* National Sleep Foundation. https://www.sleepfoundation.org/shift-work-disorder/relaxation-exercises-falling-asleep

National Sleep Foundation. (n.d.). *Sleep Patterns: Normal vs Abnormal.* Sleep Foundation. https://www.sleepfoundation.org/how-sleep-works/sleep-patterns

NIH. (2013). *The Benefits of Slumber.* NIH News in Health. https://newsinhealth.nih.gov/2013/04/benefits-slumber#:~:text=%E2%80%9CSleep%20affects%20almost%20every%20tissu

Pacheco, D. (2020, December 10). Children and Sleep.

Retrieved January 12, 2021, from https://www.sleep-foundation.org/children-and-sleep

Pagel, J. F. (2009). *Excessive Daytime Sleepiness.* American Family Physician, 79(5), 391–396. https://www.aafp.org/afp/2009/0301/p391.html

Penn Medicine. (2018, January 8). *Can You Kiss and Hug Your Way to Better Health? Research Says Yes. – Penn Medicine.* – Penn Medicine. https://www.penn-medicine.org/updates/blogs/health-and-wellness/2018/february/affection.

Petre, A. (2020, August 7). *9 Natural Sleep Aids That May Help You Get Some Shut-Eye.* Healthline. https://www.healthline.com/nutrition/sleep-aids

Rogers, A. (2008). *Sleep and Health, Need Sleep.* Harvard.Edu. http://healthysleep.med.harvard.edu/need-sleep/whats-in-it-for-you/health

Saal, K. (2019, February 19). *What is Vinyasa Yoga?: Vinyasa Flow Yoga Explained.* One Flow Yoga. https://oneflowyoga.com/blog/what-is-vinyasa-yoga.

Sleep.org. (2020, August 6). *How to Choose a Mattress.* Sleep.org. https://www.sleep.org/how-to-choose-a-mattress/.

Smith, Y. (2018, August 23). *Function of Sleep.* News-

Medical.net. https://www.news-medical.net/health/Function-of-Sleep.aspx

Suni, E. (2020, August 14). Sleepwalking - Causes, Symptoms, & Treatments. Retrieved January 12, 2021, from https://www.sleepfoundation.org/parasomnias/sleepwalking

Suni, E. (2020, November 19). *Sleep & Immunity: Can a Lack of Sleep Make You Sick?* Sleep Foundation. https://www.sleepfoundation.org/physical-health/how-sleep-affects-immunity

Suni, E. (2020, September 17). *Stress and Insomnia.* Sleep Foundation. https://www.sleepfoundation.org/insomnia/stress-and-insomnia.

Suni, E. (2020, September 25). *What is Circadian Rhythm?* Sleep Foundation. https://www.sleepfoundation.org/circadian-rhythm

The Lung Association. (2020, December 16). *Sleep Apnea.* https://www.lung.ca/lung-health/lung-disease/sleep-apnea.

Webster, M. (2008, May 6). *Can You Catch Up on Lost Sleep?* Scientific American. https://www.scientificamerican.com/article/fact-or-fiction-can-you-catch-up-on-sleep/